Living with Asperger syndrome and autism in Ireland

A book for people from adolescence to adulthood who are living with autism spectrum disorder in Ireland

by Stuart Neilson and Diarmuid Heffernan

Neilson, Stuart and Heffernan, Diarmuid

Living with Asperger syndrome and autism in Ireland / Stuart Neilson and Diarmuid Heffernan

1. HEALTH & FITNESS / Healthy Living. 2. SELF-HELP / General. 3. FAMILY & RELATIONSHIPS / Autism Spectrum Disorders.

ISBN-13: 978-1493537198
ISBN-10: 1493537199

www.autismspace.ie

v1.0

We are grateful to Aspect and the Cork Association for Autism, and to the Centre for Adult Continuing Education at Univerity College Cork for their support and advice. We would like to thank our families, especially Seán and Kit Heffernan, Siobhán Cronin and Chryssa Dislis.

Table of Contents

Table of Contents

Table of Contents

Table of Contents

Table of Contents

Table of Contents

Introduction

Welcome to this book about life with autism in Ireland. You are probably reading this far because you have been diagnosed with a label on the autism spectrum, suspect that you may have some degree of autism or have an interest because you live with or have a friendship with someone who has, or might have, an autism spectrum disorder. The term 'autistic' in this book refers to all people with autism, whether with Asperger syndrome, high-functioning autism or any other position on the spectrum. The important criterion is that the issues in your daily life relate to the issues discussed here — within the book we use the term as little as possible, just as humans exploring the moon or the ocean depths would not discuss the 'problem' of being human in those environments.

Why specifically "in Ireland"? Because this book is about life, not about autism, and we want to refer to the services, bureaucracy, social settings and other influences that create problems in everybody's life. A lot of this is very specific to the country we live in and the organisations that we have to deal with.

We also try to gather, in one place, a comprehensive reference to relevant organisations, charities, services and resources related to autism in Ireland. This includes a broad selection of books, websites and other places where you might seek more information, and refer to these where relevant in the main text. We have included our own reviews of fictional accounts of characters on the autism spectrum in film, television and books — you may find some characters you can identify with and others who are plainly nothing like you, and might use them to open up conversations about your experiences with friends or partners, or simply keep them as personal role models.

This book fills a niche not currently served in that it provides practical advice for people on the autism spectrum in an Irish context.

Outline of the book

This is a book primarily about life with autism spectrum disorder, in which life comes first and autism second — it is written, as far as possible, from the perspective of people with autism spectrum disorder and describes what life is like. This book is not full of medical descriptions (there are plenty of books that are) and does not treat autism as 'a problem', although we begin with a description of autism spectrum disorder in **Chapter 1**. We relegate the rest of the medical material to the back of the book, but if you are in the position of being undiagnosed but suspecting that you may have an autism spectrum disorder, then you might want to skip ahead to **Chapter 10** for information about recognizing autism. We also discuss the process of diagnosis, the pros and cons of getting yourself labelled as having autism and a description of the main routes to diagnosis in Ireland in **Chapter 11**. We finish off the book with **Chapter 12** describing current research and issues in autism spectrum disorder, including debates about diagnosis, causes and the changing frequency of autism. We also describe advances in screening and testing people, including MRI scans and more common questionnaire and observational tests.

Throughout the book there are references to organisations, websites, other books and media. We have collected everything together in the **Appendices**, where you will find a directory of groups, services, websites and resources related to autism spectrum disorder. It can be dipped into whenever necessary for fuller details about organisations that are referred to in the text, or in response to any issue that arises in your own life. We have also included a short review of many films, books and TV series that have representations of people with autism, which might be the common reference that many people have for what autism is, or might be a model that you can use when describing your own experiences.

In **Chapter 2**, we talk about day-to-day issues that affect us all, such as sensory sensitivities, anxiety, mood and meltdowns (and how to cope with the embarrassment afterwards). We also talk about common self-care issues like dealing with illness, handling intimate questions and communicating about ill-health or emotion.

We discuss the benefits of a wide range of drugs (both legal and illegal, over-the-counter and prescribed) and food supplements that people commonly use.

In **Chapter 3** we discuss relationships, principally relationships outside your own family, although we touch on that too. We discuss how anxiety and sensory issues can impact on dealing with strangers, or with people you meet in unfamiliar places, such as shopping or (if that is your inclination) night-clubbing. We also discuss how to recognize friendship or hostility in other people, and how general people-centred skills might be developed, along with the lifelong, routine business of maintaining friendships and acquaintances over time. We also discuss issues of identity (such as fashion and membership of groups), sexuality and the social pressures to be in a couple. Not forgetting sex itself, with that wonderful mixture of pleasant and frightening sensations, and developing trust with a partner.

We lump school, college and work together in **Chapter 4**, because (in Western society, at least) our schools are miniature models of the work environment, designed to train new generations of producer-consumer into compliance and conformity. The problems of being in a rigid, hierarchical, rule-based system can be a great comfort to some people who like predictability and order, and a huge burden on people who rebel against uniformity. We discuss issues of bullying, using rules to your advantage and issues about being different. We also discuss college entry, job interviews and working in a team.

Planning work, study and activities is a common problem for many people, often blocked by anxiety, the complexity of unknowable outcomes, lack of motivation and unattainable perfectionism. In **Chapter 5** we describe useful techniques for managing time and resources. We use a variety of paper-based planning, technological solutions, mood management exercises and personal training.

Activities of daily living include the obvious cleaning, cooking and washing, as well as personal hygiene and self-care. A lot of these issues are 'obvious' things that can become very difficult as people grow up, change household, start to live alone or start living with someone else. We discuss issues like managing a wardrobe, shopping and catering for social groups. We conclude **Chapter 6** by looking at how to find help with activities of daily living when they become too difficult to handle, and with how to recognize when you are not coping with everyday activities and need help.

Once someone has a diagnosis (of anything, not just autism) it is quite common that everything — mood, bodily discomfort or pain, poor concentration — is attributed to that one diagnosis, by family, friends and even by doctors. People with autism spectrum disorder become ill and have health problems just like every other person, and in **Chapter 7** we talk about medical issues that are not part of autism spectrum disorder, how to differentiate which symptoms or behaviours might be something else and how to communicate these issues to a doctor, particularly when a doctor might be dismissive of symptoms that could be confused with autism. One issue of particular concern is the development of psychiatric illness (such as depression) that is both brought on by anxiety and sensory stress, and presents symptoms of emotional under-responsiveness and social withdrawal — in other words both generated by and mimicking autistic behaviour.

In **Chapter 8** we talk about managing barriers to getting things done. Money and bureaucracy are issues that can be ignored when things are going well, but become very serious when things are not going well. The most important theme we build is the need to deal with finances and bureaucracy in good time, which is to say the earlier the better. The same applies whether it is returning job applications, getting a passport, dealing with parking fines or dealing with tax returns. No matter how unpleasant they are, the unpleasantness is minimized when the issue is handled in good time. We also discuss social welfare and disability-related entitlements.

Chapter 9 is largely motivated by hearing someone ask "What can someone with autism do?", as if somehow the entire horizon of life expectations is entirely different, or foreshortened, by autism. Children with autism spectrum disorder dream of being astronauts, vets, nurses or sexy actors, just like any other child. And, just like any other child, they will (almost all) discover a growing gap between the reality and the childhood fantasy, which is entirely normal. We discuss growing up, education, the transition from school to college or employment, relationships and lifetime achievement, and how to align effort or achievement with aspiration.

In **Chapter 10** we look at ways of recognizing traits of autism in yourself or in those close to you. We begin by challenging the idea of 'normal' before looking at practical ways of developing your own self awareness. The central part of this chapter describes scenarios, experiences and online screening tests which may help in recognizing autism traits. We finish the chapter by describing how a loved one or friend may begin the conversation with someone they feel may have an autism spectrum disorder, and how this conversation may be helped by the raising of public awareness of autism.

In **Chapter 11** we discuss the pros and cons of getting a diagnosis of autism. We look at some of the potential benefits such as access to early interventions, supports in primary, second level and third level education as well as 'disability' social welfare payments. We then look at the potential negative outcomes of diagnosis such as stigma, bullying and stereotyping. We discuss the idea of autism as being a difference or a disability before finishing with a how-to guide on getting diagnosed in Ireland.

In **Chapter 12** we delve into current research and debate about the autism spectrum, beginning with a discussion of the controversial new fifth edition of the DSM. We also look at the link between genetics and autism as well as the use of MRI scans to detect autism. We conclude this chapter by describing the Autism Bill in Ireland, the portrayal of autism spectrum disorders in the media and the future for people with autism spectrum disorders in Ireland.

The appendices include brief reviews of books, television series and films that feature a principle character with autism in **Appendix A**, a list of further reading books and websites in **Appendix B**, full contact details of organisations useful to people living with autism in Ireland in **Appendix C** and a glossary of useful terms and abbreviations in **Appendix D**.

1 What is Asperger syndrome? (Diarmuid Heffernan)

We will begin with a number of scenarios which may sound familiar to you. For example: perhaps you make more social faux-pas than other people (people without autistic spectrum disorders will be referred to as the neurologically typical or neurotypicals throughout this book) and still don't understand them when they are explained to you, perhaps you often feel stressed and anxious when you are in public spaces, or you feel that you become irrational and cannot cope with lots of noise and activity, perhaps you feel that other people seem to have a knowledge and understanding of social mores (a common social language that you don't understand). If some or indeed all of these scenarios sound familiar to you then this book is for you. We will begin this chapter by exploring some definitions of Asperger syndrome and interspersing it with how this may relate to you. We try to use reader friendly language as much as possible in the chapter but some technical terminology is unavoidable (and probably best read in the context of this book which sets out to be as non medicalised as possible).

Asperger syndrome (AS) is a condition on the autistic spectrum. It is easiest to think of the autistic spectrum as an arc with Asperger syndrome on this arc with many other points along the way which make up the diverse nature, characteristics and experience of human beings on the Autism Spectrum. AS is generally categorised as being an autistic spectrum disorder (ASD). Much of what has been written and researched about AS has been subsumed into general ASD research. In addition the term AS has been subsumed into ASD without separate status in the fifth edition of the Diagnostic and Statistical Manual of Mental Disorders (DSM-5), hence in this text the focus will be on AS but the terms AS and ASD will be used interchangeably. The Diagnostic and Statistical Manual of Mental Disorders, fifth edition is published by the American Psychiatric Association and is one of a number of diagnostic frameworks used in Ireland. The DSM sets out all conditions that fall into the category of mental disorder. The

DSM-5 has subsumed AS into the ASD categorisation as there are question marks as to its separate status. This may have a profound effect on you if you decide to seek a diagnosis (see chapter 11) as it means that the services which provide support for people with Asperger syndrome may have their funding affected. This is because each HSE area receives a finite amount of funding. There is a big difference in the amount of funding needed for a residential service for people with autism requiring twenty four hour staffing and for example an outreach service for people with Asperger syndrome. If there is no distinction made between Asperger syndrome and autism there may therefore be consequences for services which are specific to Asperger syndrome as their funding may be subsumed into the need for residential funding. A further issue in terms of the proposed change by the DSM is the issue of identity. For many people on the spectrum the Asperger identity is an important one in that it is a community, a way of providing explanation for ways of thinking, it is not prescriptive but it does offer a framework of understanding for different ways of thinking or being. We discuss the ramifications of the new DSM in greater detail in chapter 12.

1.1 Defining Asperger syndrome

There is ongoing debate and controversy as to the definition of AS. AS has been variously described and defined since the condition was first discovered by Austrian Paediatrician Hans Asperger in 1944. It is a condition on the Autistic Spectrum and is clinically classed as a pervasive developmental disorder. As mentioned in the introduction, Asperger syndrome is on what is called the autistic spectrum and is therefore referred to as an autistic spectrum disorder. "Autistic Spectrum Disorders" (or ASD's) essentially describes all types of autism and places them on an autistic spectrum.

This spectrum runs from profound autism at one side, to high functioning autism or Asperger syndrome at the other. The best and possibly simplest way of describing Asperger syndrome is to look at the differences you may feel you have compared to other people. For example a difference in social imagination, how other people seem to have a supernatural ability to read each other's intent, how they seem to be able to adapt so easily to change/different environments/ new routines or social situations, how others seem to react irrationally to your statements of factual reality (yes that dress does look awful on you!), how others act like noise/odour/small nuclear explosions don't bother them! These experiences may be broadly categorised under the so called triad of impairments which are social impairments in: interaction, communication and imagination. There are no definitive causes of Asperger syndrome although many reasons have been put forward including genetics. There is even a theory that relates the condition to an adaptation to the technological age we now live in, and people with ASDs may in fact represent the next step in human evolution! Neurobiological research has narrowed down the differences between the brain of someone with AS from neurotypicals to neurological differences with, for example, difference in the amygdala and cerebellum and difference in functioning in the right cortical hemisphere. What this means in essence is that the 'social' parts of the brain function differently than in neurotypicals, so next time you are having difficulty reading a social cue just remember that you have a brain that works differently from those who appear to inherently understand social mores. MRI scans also show differences between Asperger syndrome and autism.

1.2 Causes of Asperger syndrome

There has been much speculation and debate as to the causes of Asperger syndrome but what is important to remember is to be selective of the sources of information around autistic spectrum disorders you use, as much of what is put on the internet in particular is unsubstantiated. We will adhere to what is factually and scientifically known in this section. Hans Asperger, had originally conducted a study on four socially awkward children who seemed to have difficulty relating to others and had a narrow focus of interests based on specific topics. Asperger used the term 'autism' which came from literature on schizophrenia to describe their condition. This term had originally been used the previous year by Leo Kanner (1943) who is the first person to research autism (the word autism comes from 'autos' meaning 'self' in Greek and refers to the sense of people with autism being 'locked in'). Asperger's research had been written in German and because papers written in German were very much frowned upon in Europe and America subsequent to the second World War. This was because of the association with Nazism, eugenics and experimentation on humans. Therefore it had lain dormant until British Psychiatrist Lorna Wing published an article in 1981 which first applied the term Asperger syndrome to some 34 patients she was working with.

This article also lay dormant and was not picked up on by either the medical or research fields. In fact it took another ten years until Uta Frith published a book called "Autism and Asperger syndrome" before the medical community began to take notice. This was confirmed in 1994 when the American Psychiatric Association and the World Health Organisation included Asperger syndrome in the diagnostic classification system of medical conditions and it was included in both the DSM and ICD.

1.3 Diagnostic systems

Although research is ongoing with significant debate on the primary characteristics of Asperger syndrome, the characteristics generally used to clinically define the condition are social awkwardness and difficulty relating to others, failure to develop peer relationships, unusual use and type of language, a lack of empathy (please note that this is a contentious and ambiguous term and may be more accurate to describe it as an impaired ability to recognise emotions correctly, inability to properly read social cues and facial expressions, anxiety, bluntness, narrow interests and repetitive actions). These characteristics however are among a variety of different personality aspects that make up the clinical diagnosis of Asperger syndrome and therefore you may read this and think I don't fit all of the criteria as set out. If you should choose to explore getting a diagnosis please bear this in mind. It is important to note at this point that AS is characterised as a disjunctive category in that no two people with AS necessarily share the same diagnostic symptoms. It is also important to note that that vast complex tapestry of experiences that every human being experiences may impact on any set of diagnostic criteria used. There is therefore much debate on both the criteria used to diagnose and indeed the defining characteristics of Asperger syndrome.

1.4 DSM and ICD

If you do choose to explore the possibility of getting a diagnosis then there are two main references for descriptive or diagnostic criteria for Asperger syndrome. They are the Diagnostic and Statistical Manual of Mental Disorders (DSM), and the International Classification of Diseases (ICD). Both books are very similar in their criteria for definition of Asperger syndrome. The DSM of the American Psychiatric Association Diagnostic Criteria for Asperger syndrome is the most commonly used diagnostic tool in the United States while the ICD tends to used more frequently in the United Kingdom (NAS, 2013). The DSM-5 has recently been published and has generated much debate (we discuss this in more detail in chapter 12) as it has changed the diagnostic criteria for Asperger syndrome from the previously used DSM-IV. The American Psychiatric Association (APA) researched the new diagnostic criteria for a decade at an estimated cost of 20-25 million dollars which they say came from their own reserves. The Manual has changed the criteria for diagnosis of ASD from three main criteria based on the Triad of Impairments to two main criteria — in the DSM-IV these were impairments in communication, social interaction and restricted interests and repetitive behaviours, in the new DSM-5 the communication and social interaction criteria are combined based on social/communication difficulties. The APA say that the DSM-5 criteria has subsumed four different disorders — Autistic Disorder, Asperger's Disorder, Childhood Disintegrative Disorder and Pervasive Developmental Disorder Not Otherwise Specified (PDD-NOS) into one category — ASD. The association believes that this is a "better reflection of the state of knowledge about autism ... a single umbrella disorder will improve the diagnosis of ASD without limiting the sensitivity of the criteria, or substantially changing the number of children being diagnosed" (APA, 2013). The new criteria also aim to address the fact that the "symptoms of people with ASD will fall on a continuum, with some individuals showing mild symptoms and others having much more severe symptoms. This spectrum will allow clinicians to account for the variations in symptoms and behaviours from person to person ... under the DSM-5 criteria, individuals with ASD must show symptoms from early childhood, even if those symptoms are not recognized until later ... this allows people whose symptoms may not be fully recognized until social demands exceed their capacity to receive the diagnosis. It is an important change from DSM-IV criteria, which was geared toward identifying school-aged children with autism-related disorders, but not as useful in diagnosing younger children" (APA, 2013). Sensory behaviours are included in the criteria of the DSM-5 for the first time, under the 'restricted, repetitive patterns of behaviours'. The DSM-5 has also included what it terms 'dimensional elements' which give an indication of how much someone's condition affects them. This will help to identify how much support an individual needs. The APA has also created a new diagnosis called Social Communication Disorder. This is characterised by difficulties with verbal and non-verbal communication that cannot be explained by low cognitive ability (NAS, 2013).

1.5 The Gillberg diagnostic criteria

Another commonly used diagnostic assessment tool is one devised by Christopher Gillberg in 1991 which is closely based on Hans Asperger's original diagnostic criteria, and centres on impairments in social interaction, impositions of routines, speech and language problems and motor clumsiness.

1.6 How do I know if I have Asperger syndrome?

Should you choose to explore getting a diagnosis there are a few routes for yourself, family member, child etc. One way is to begin by approaching your G.P. and asking for a referral to either a psychiatrist or psychologist who specialise in the diagnosis of Asperger syndrome. The other way is to make an appointment directly with a psychiatrist or psychologist yourself. There is a useful guide in the Appendices of this book as to services/diagnosticians in your local area. If you would prefer to do an online test (which we must stress is not a substitute for a clinical diagnosis) there are some useful websites which are included in the appendices.

1.7 Prevalence

You may be interested to discover that there are ever increasing numbers of people diagnosed with an autistic spectrum disorder (there has been much talk of an explosion of ASDs and much debate around the reasons for this but in this text we will stick with reputable sources of information and thus remain as factually based as possible). There are varying estimates of the number of people with ASDs and indeed it is difficult to pin down the number because ASD remains a diagnosis that is defined behaviourally and with the opinion of the medical professional carrying out the diagnosis, as well as the fact that diagnostic assessment is complex and expensive. Current figures from the National Autistic Society in the UK estimate that 1% of the population have ASDs.

This figure has risen due to greater awareness of ASDs amongst the public and professionals. Figures for those with AS are much more difficult to calculate as these tend to be subsumed into overall ASD figures. Ehlers and Gillberg estimate the rate to be between one in 210 to one in 280 (this translates as 0.3-0.5% of the population) although Tony Attwood feels that only fifty percent of children with Asperger syndrome are now being diagnosed. It does appear however that there have been huge increases in the numbers of people receiving diagnosis in the last ten years. There has been much speculation about the reasons for this increase, but greater awareness of ASDs amongst relevant professionals and society at large is seen as being a vital contributory factor. In line with increased diagnosis and awareness there is also a growing presence of people with AS who are representing themselves through literature and other forums.

1.8 Differing Prevalence between males and females

There is a difference in numbers of males compared to females being diagnosed with AS. Some put the difference as high as 1 woman to every four men being diagnosed. This difference has been linked by some to a male genetic factor. Others however surmise that it may have something to do with a female ability to 'mask' the difficulties associated with AS a bit better. This may be problematic for many women as the ability to hide the difficulties associated with AS may not mean that they experience less distress and in some cases may increase distress because of masking it. Furthermore some feel it may be because women have a better developed sense of empathy and therefore are more likely to be accepting of difference in those with AS.

1.9 Neurodiversity

The term neurodiversity is credited to AS parent Judy Singer who first spoke of a "neurological diversity, or what I want to call Neurodiversity". The term and the concept were then taken on by support groups and online lobby groups, for example (www.neurodiversity.com) to advance the notion of difference rather than disability. This concept has as its core the fundamental belief that human beings exist on a continuum where various behaviours and ways of looking at the world exist.

Rather than looking at how any person or group exists in terms of what is deemed to be normal, the lobby calls for differences to be recognised and acknowledged as opposed to being stigmatised and viewed as aberrant. This notion has significant consequences for all who are viewed as disabled and many feel it may help revolutionize the way we look at mental health. While people with ASDs are framed in terms of being on a spectrum, the neurodiversity movement regards all human beings as being on a spectrum of biological, cognitive and neurological diversity, whether they have a diagnosis of an ASD or not.

In many ways the neurodiversity movement is also a response to current research, one strand of which has examined the potential for detecting autism in the womb. This potential new test would mean that by testing the levels of testosterone in the amniotic fluid that autism may be detectable in the womb and therefore would give parents the choice to proceed with the pregnancy or to terminate it. This is essentially pre-emptive 'curing' and would be viewed by many as a great break through for the medical profession. Many others however feel that it would question what kind of society and world we would like to live in, and question the very right to existence of people on the autistic spectrum. Writing on this subject in the Guardian newspaper Simon Baron-Cohen sums up this view: "if there was a prenatal test for autism would this be desirable? What would you lose if children with autism spectrum disorders were eliminated from the population?"

In answer to this question and in direct contrast to the argument for pre-emptive curing, there has been research compiled around the possibility of ASDs representing an evolutionary step forward. This work has been spearheaded by Simon Baron-Cohen who has looked at the propensity for many on the autistic spectrum to prefer, and be particularly skilled at, interaction with computers. A prominent example of these skills is Bram Cohen the inventor of the Torrents file sharing system, and person with AS. Baron-Cohen's work has included studies on Silicon Valley where prevalence rates for ASDs are particularly high as previously mentioned (there is speculation that AS people prefer to have AS partners and assortative mating is the cause of high Silicon Valley child autism prevalence). This has led to a theory that given the increased interface between humans and computers that people with ASDs either represent an evolutionary step forward to adapt to our IT world, or, given the fact that our world is hugely reliant on IT, that people with ASDs will prove invaluable in the human-IT nexus.

There is however, much criticism of the neurodiversity movement from without and within the ASD community (such that a community exists in a hugely diverse and heterogeneous group). Much of the criticism is expressed in online forums and proposes that neurodiversity does not acknowledge the individual difficulties faced by people with ASDs which may be disabling. A further criticism focuses largely on the fact that the neurodiversity movement is representative of a distinct subset within the ASD spectrum. This subset is a particularly vocal and articulate group within the ASD community who do not represent the views of all on the spectrum but rather the more 'able' individuals on it (www.autisminnb.blogspot.com).

Something which you may relate to in your own life is the fact that one of the distinguishing characteristics of autism in the public consciousness is a sense that those with the condition are 'odd' or not 'normal' (see for example the portrayal of a man with autism in the movie "Rainman"). This has meant that many people with autism feel excluded in public spaces. The neurodiversity movement calls for understanding and acceptance from the dominant 'neurotypical' community to understand the neurological differences of AS that may manifest in 'unusual' or 'abnormal' behaviour in public spaces.

This 'unusual' behaviour has been addressed by early intervention models such as Applied Behaviour Analysis (ABA) which sets out to identify behaviours that are deemed unacceptable (but which you may find reassuring or relaxing particularly in stressful social situations) such as stimming, and to positively reinforce behaviours that are deemed apposite such as appropriate social interaction. In its essence ABA teaches ASD children to behave 'normally' through a positive reward system which is predicated on learnt behaviours. It does not allow for the differences that neurodiversity celebrates but rather takes as its starting point an agreed societal version of the 'norm' which AS children are taught to adhere to. An example of this is in the "Handbook for Parent Training" which proposes denying a child with an ASD food until they make sufficient eye contact to satisfy the parent (pg 75). This example, while undoubtedly well-meaning, may be contrasted with Florica Stone's example in "Autism — The Eight Colour of The Rainbow" which suggests that many children on the spectrum may not be able to focus on two things at once, so if they are being asked to look at a parent and eat food, or if, for example, there is a sensory stimulus occurring in the room, that the child may be unable to focus on the parent. Stone in this book advises creating a connection with the child and understanding what he or she may be finding difficult and adjusting your parental response and inputs accordingly. A further criticism of ABA is that it teaches AS children to act 'normally' as opposed to understanding why they are behaving differently to their classmates. It also teaches children to 'act' normally, without taking into account the possibility that these children are acting as they are told without having any understanding of why they have to act in this way. Acting 'normal' in this way may also be obvious to others and they may see it as being obvious as learnt normal behaviour. This performance of normality may be exhausting and confusing for many with ASDs, particularly in public spaces. This is not to say that ABA is anything other than well meaning or indeed that parents don't report great satisfaction with the program. Many feel it has been hugely beneficial for their children and in recent years there has been (thus far) unresearched reports of children 'losing' the symptoms of Autism.

1.10 Asperger syndrome and the internet

One space in which those who have been diagnosed with AS have chosen to express themselves is through the internet. This has been manifest through the previously explored neurodiversity movement but is also evident in the number of online forums run by and for people with AS. The internet serves as a virtual podium for many with AS who feel insecure or unable to express themselves in face to face or traditional ways. The virtual space of the internet represents a facility which simplifies interaction and communication. It replaces the social norms, the expectations and the rules which may be confusing for some people with AS, with a different set of expectations where issues of, for example, body language, intonation or emotional vibes are not part of the medium. It reduces communication to its most pure and simple form without the implicit difficulties that public or social interaction may create.

In light of the increased prevalence of technology and particularly use of the internet in the daily lives of many of us, the opportunities to communicate in this way have grown exponentially. It is also a manifestation of the individualisation of communication and the prevalence amongst people generally, regardless of having AS or not, to communicate via the internet. As previously stated the internet provides dual opportunities as a safe space of communication for those with AS, and also represents a forum for people with AS to represent themselves.

The internet may be seen in many ways as a modern day platform by which civil society engages and debates, the contemporary equivalent of the cafés in which civil society initially began to express itself. Many people with AS argue that their condition is merely a difference in neurological functioning and therefore a variance on what it is to be human. The internet provides a space by which this opinion may be disseminated.

The logical nature of technology also suits many with AS. It has a system and a logical way of operating that in some ways echoes the qualities of many with AS. The predictability of the interaction between the (AS) person and computer is soothing and contrasts with the unpredictability of 'neurotypical' people. Many with AS also use internet gaming as a way by which to express themselves and create an alternate cyber-reality that makes more sense to them than the lived reality. For example online games such as "World of Warcraft" or "Minecraft" have shared rules which all adhere to and understand. In the space represented by cyber-reality the person is in control, rules are obvious and each action has a reaction and a consequence, there is no judgement and no expectation, which may contrast greatly with the experience of many with AS in public spaces.

This is not to say that everyone with AS necessarily uses the internet as a means to represent their views or indeed to interact with others. Many with AS would rather communicate face to face with others and reject the use of the internet for this purpose. This view is indicative of the great diversity that exists within the AS community. For some the internet represents a safe space of communication and a platform for their views. For others it is just a practical tool by which to perform functional tasks.

Despite the claim of Judy Singer that the internet represents a "democratization of information flow" which has created a new way for people with ASDs to represent their identities, the internet is also unbounded in terms of the content that can be accessed and disseminated through it. The democratic and free speech nature of the internet allows for every opinion about ASDs to be posted and this runs the gamut from helpful forums to false and damaging claims about ASDs.

Therefore the internet may be used by some with AS to positively inform people about the condition and to raise public awareness, but it may also be a source of inaccurate or false information. The gradual increase in awareness of AS as a condition (as evidenced for example by a major TV series made about the life of Temple Grandin) has led to increased content on the internet being written about AS. This has been very varied with positive stories such as those written about the remarkable skills of autistic woman

Amanda Baggs to the numerous entries around AS and its link with various forms of deviance. So while the internet may be a space of safety, expression and freedom for some, it also simultaneously exists as a site of judgement and misinformation which may reflect some of the very views that make public spaces so uncomfortable for many with AS. Our advice is to tread carefully, the internet is a useful tool and a potentially less stressful alternative to interacting face to face but it is also mirrors many of the bad aspects in society generally and if an individual places too much emphasis on interacting through the virtual world there are many inherent potential difficulties which may make it as difficult as face to face interaction. This is evidenced in the ongoing discourse around cyber-bullying and the many individual cases of online bullying and victimisation. The propensity for many people to view the virtual world as being a medium where there are no consequences to their actions also needs to be fully researched but as time goes by and more evidence of this exists, it is wise to weigh this up when considering ways of interacting with others.

1.11 School, family and society

As explored in other parts of this book, getting or having a diagnosis of Asperger syndrome has a number of different sides to it. On the one hand the idea of having a label can be unappealing and potentially stigmatising, while on the other it provides an explanation for all those ways in your life that you feel differently to others. For many, receiving a diagnosis means experiencing all of the above emotions and many others simultaneously. But what does it mean to feel different in school, family or society generally?

1.12 School

School is the first real public space in which the majority of us interact, and where comparisons are made between us and others. Of course we interact with our families and with friends etc before we attend school but school involves more intense interactions with many people you don't know, may not understand or don't like. Primary school is a space which is fraught with potential difficulties such as: I don't want to play with the other children as they are playing a game I am not interested in, I want to play by myself and the teachers are telling me I must play and share with the other children. This requires negotiation and learning on your part in terms of how you interact with others and how you make your passage through school easier. Finding your niche in school usually involves finding someone else (or a few others) who are interested in the same things as you are. So for example if you love fighter planes or history or playing computer games then finding someone else who has the same interests can be very useful in making your path through school easier. You may also find the routine and rigour of school is helpful if not enjoyable. The set times of classes and the set routines of certain classrooms at certain times can be reassuring.

Secondary school may potentially bring a different set of problems. It is usually bigger than primary school and it is also likely that in primary school you may not feel, or may not be treated very differently from other children even if you do things differently than others. This is because younger children tend not to notice differences between each other at a younger age, they are generally more naive and are more likely to be openly curious and ask why you have done or said something different rather than to judge it. In secondary school however, adolescents become more likely to notice and potentially exploit difference. There are a number of reasons for this including trying to fit in, the nature of hierarchy, and hormonal changes. The need to find a place in the social pecking order is often done at the expense of others. In other words bullying or picking on others is a way of fitting in and for many people who do it, it masks their own insecurities and fears. So secondary school is a time which is fraught with many issues and areas of concern for all teenagers and especially those who may feel or act differently or who find it difficult to understand the social expectations of school. On the other hand school rules as mentioned previously may be reassuring. For the most part difference can cause difficulties in school. However, difference in thinking, adherence to routine and enjoying certain subjects can be to your advantage in terms of surviving school and performing academically. It may also work to your advantage to be interested in certain niche subjects as members of the opposite, or same, sex may see this as being attractive. Maybe being the mysterious outsider might give you some cache or make you appear cool and sophisticated to others (you should already know that you are cool anyway — how many other kids can claim to genuinely have a different way of looking at things without it being a stance designed to make them appear cool!).

1.13 Your family

Families have to be survived. As Oliver James intriguingly titled book suggests "They f*** you up". Families can represent a bastion of safety and reassurance, they can be your best (or sometimes only) friends. They may make more effort than anyone else in your life to understand your perspective. They may forgive you when you tell Aunt Gertrude to her face that she is a snob and she smells like mothballs. They may be extremely proud of you when you ace your school exams, or they may go miles out their way to drive you to that building that Frank Gehry designed. On the other hand they may shout at you when you refuse to take out the bins as it is not your turn, or get angry and embarrassed when you tell your Aunt Gertude she is a snob and smells like mothballs!

Families represent micro social systems that are a complex sum of their parts. They are formed by a unique set of variables and are thus unique in their construction and in their interactions and inter-relations. You may find it difficult to get on with your siblings as they may not understand your perspective — or you theirs. However it is worthwhile trying to find a common ground with your family. They can be very helpful and supportive to you and doing your best to try and negotiate with them can make for a more harmonious family home. The best way of doing this is by sitting down with them and explaining that you are not being unhelpful or nasty, but rather you see things in a particular way. Rather than either you or your family becoming entrenched in certain positions you should all be open in describing what you may find difficult to do or understand. This openness is difficult to do for everyone but is worth taking the risk on.

There are many other practical steps that you may employ in order to have a better relationship with your family and them with you. One of these steps is to give each other space, both physical and emotional. If you have found it difficult over the years to express yourself or to understand family member's point of view, then it may have created divisions and tensions between you. These are not easily remedied but communication is the first step to any successful relationship — be it friendship, romantic relationship or family. Saying to your family that you need space (and explaining why) may relieve some of the tension that may have built up, and often times the creation of a physical space can allow objectivity to occur and possibly a better understanding of issues from each perspective. This can be especially true for people who have not yet been diagnosed. Many people with AS have reported a change and improvement in family relationships after being diagnosed as their families have a greater understanding of the diagnosed individual's perspective. In many cases the desires and wishes that families may have for each other are simply that — their own desires and wishes and they may not tally with the desires or needs of someone with AS. This dissonance is often at the centre of family tensions. It must be said however that getting a diagnosis is not a panacea and many people with AS still have difficulties with their families post diagnosis especially when families do not accept the diagnosis or even the existence of AS.

If you are still living at home as an adult, then it may be worth looking into independent housing options. This may be dependent on whether you are employed, your income or the type of welfare payment you are in receipt of if you are unemployed. There are social housing associations who provide low cost housing options and given the current economic situation there are also many rental accommodation options. The advantages of living independently are myriad — such as increasing your confidence, and increasing your repertoire of living skills, but in the context of your relationship with your family you may find that having your own space may improve interactions radically.

1.14 Society

The principles of coping with school and negotiating with your family also apply to society generally. We all must find our own way, niche and path in life and this is not an easy journey for anyone. The journey of life runs the gamut from the naivety and fear of childhood to the confusion of adolescence before transitioning to the responsibility of adulthood and all that it entails. Society is increasingly influenced by the Western capitalist consumerist model that the Irish state appears to have embraced whole heartedly. This involves the view of citizens — from the state's perspective — as potential economic contributors, tax payers, as automatons in the various multi-national machines that we appear to be more and more reliant on. So what does this mean for you? Well, you are at an advantage, in that you think differently from many of the people around you and certainly most of the people who run the country! You may be able to avoid the pitfalls of group-think, you potentially have a unique perspective on things and you frequently have a strong social conscience. So in dealing with others in society generally, while you have many advantageous and enviable qualities, there are some social etiquettes you should be aware of. For example giving your honest opinion is a fantastic trait that is all too rare in our modern world, however try to bear in mind that there is a line beyond which honesty may become hurtful. For instance, you may think the painting your mother/brother/friend etc asks you to comment on is awful, try to find the positives in it, you are not lying but rather you are showing emotional intelligence and maturity and a regard for the other persons feelings. So you might for example say "I would not be able to paint that and how did you get those brush strokes to look like that — it's very impressive and interesting".

It is important to say that there is growing awareness of autism spectrum disorders generally in society. The media have been very influential in this shift through movies and in the many books discussing the topic — including this one! There has been a gradual paradigm shift from the types of stereotypical representations of people with autism, see for example the movie "Rainman" to movies such as "Adam" which many feel are more representative of the diversity of the autism spectrum.

In public spaces there may be things you do to calm your anxieties such as flapping your arms or talking to yourself to reassure yourself. We think it best to be aware that if you do things that are deemed out of the ordinary by others then you may draw unwanted attention on yourself. This is not to say you should not do it, but rather to understand that others may view it as being 'unusual' or 'odd'. If you feel that it is very difficult to be in public spaces without reassuring yourself then maybe listening to your favourite music on your headphones, or even recordings of your own voice reassuring you, might be useful, in essence, use whatever works best for you. In the next chapter we examine day-to-day issues and in the following chapter we will look at the issue of relationships with others, including interacting with strangers, what constitutes a friendship, as well as sexuality and identity.

2 Day-to-day issues *(Stuart Neilson)*

In this chapter we explore what everyday life is like with autism and how the traits and symptoms interact with everyday functioning. Along the way, we explain some methods of handling the problems that might arise for you. We also explore how some coping strategies — including some that you might have developed yourself, consciously or unconsciously — can actually limit opportunities.

We talk, in turn, about sensory issues, psychological issues, medical care and finally the effect of drugs. This order reflects the immediacy with which these things affect someone with autism — sensory issues might not be the most important issue, but, if you have sensory problems, then they are there every day, from the moment you first wake up. Managing sensory issues effectively can make a tremendous difference to everything else you do, including lessening the frequency and severity of psychological problems, and decreasing the reliance on drugs or other interventions that help.

2.1 Sensory issues

Everybody feels the world differently, and with differences in intensity. We don't even know to what degree the feelings that we share through language actually reflect shared experience, because we can never get inside another mind to experience the same senses as another person. For instance, is the sensation that I have when perceiving the colour red equal to yours? We only know that (most of the time) two people will agree to call the same colours with the same names. One of the most noticeable aspects of being on the autism spectrum is that senses do appear to be different from other people around you, and from every other person with autism. Some sensations will be more intense, often to the point of extreme discomfort, and others will be diminished causing issues like clumsiness. A further factor that is noticeable to people on the autism spectrum is that the brain processes senses differently from people around you — for instance, you might sometimes notice a delay between hearing words and those words starting to make sense, or words might make no sense at all when you are feeling under stress. Other sensory issues might include sensitivity to skin contact, acute sensitivity to unpleasant noises, a dislike of some everyday smells or difficulty coping with foods with unpleasant textures.

Interestingly, sensory issues have not been part of the International Classification of Disease (ICD) or the Diagnostic and Statistical Manual (DSM) criteria for recognizing autism spectrum disorder, even though they are common in people with autism spectrum disorder. Sensory issues are included for the first time in DSM-5 as another aspect of restricted and repetitive behaviours, described by "hyper- or hypo-reactivity to sensory input or unusual interest in sensory aspects of environment; (such as apparent indifference to pain / heat / cold, adverse response to specific sounds or textures, excessive smelling or touching of objects, fascination with lights or spinning objects)". Obviously, sensory issues go much further than this and underlie many other behaviours, whether it is dressing to avoid sensory exposure or experiencing a meltdown due to sensory overload in a busy or unfamiliar setting.

We will discuss noise, light, touch, food texture and smell. You might have your own issues that differ from these, but the principles are similar. Sensory exposure is something that we can not avoid in order to live a full and productive life — you can not always eliminate unpleasant senses, and sometimes the unpleasant exposure is a compromise in order to achieve something else (noise is unavoidable if you go to work, rejecting every food you do not like is bad manners). However, sensory experiences are often predictable and in many cases you can learn to either minimise their impact or to minimise your strong reactions to them. We want to promote responses to sensory difficulties that help you to overcome the problem and continue with whatever you want to do, and to encourage you not to merely avoid unpleasant sensory experiences.

Noise is constantly around us, everywhere except inside anechoic chambers (used to test sensitive measurement equipment, or design microphones) and in therapeutic flotation chambers, or isolation tanks, where you float at skin temperature in silent darkness to experience a degree of sensory deprivation. You have more control over noise at home than outside, but can rarely eliminate all the noises that bother you. Typical sources of irritating noise are fluorescent lighting (including low-energy compact fluorescent bulbs, although these have become very much quieter then when they were first available), old-style glass TV or computer screens, power transformers, traffic noise and the noises of other people's daily activities — TV, radio and work activities. Many people either do not hear or are completely unbothered by noises that you might find infuriating or upsetting. Some simple methods of controlling noise include isolation, absorption and masking. You can isolate high-frequency noises fairly easily by closing windows and doors, wearing a hat or ear-plugs and choosing to work or relax further from sources of noise. Ear-muffs or over-ear headphones (even if you are not listening to music) will decrease noise exposure at the same time as reducing potentially unpleasant wind and cold sensations on your ears — wearing larger earphones in public has become more popular in recent years due to branding like Beats and Skullcandy. One consequence of covering your ears in public is that your may increase your social isolation, either because you can not hear conversation or because other people will not speak to you because they believe that you can not hear conversation — but this might suit you in the circumstances that you choose to wear them, such as when out walking for exercise. You can absorb high frequency noises by having carpets, rugs, wall-hangings and soft furnishings to reduce sound reflections. Neither of these will deal effectively with low-frequency noises like traffic, aircraft engines or heavy machinery because of the thickness and mass of the absorbing material that would be required. Some ear protectors, used on building sites, or isolating earplugs might help, but are not comfortable for extended periods of wear. Electronic noise-cancelling headphones are also effective, but are deliberately designed not to eliminate the sounds of human voices, as a safety measure to ensure that wearers hear warnings. Finally, masking can work for some people who have a sound that is enjoyable and able to hold that part of the attention that is disturbed by environmental noises — typical sounds are music, running water or birdsong, often on a CD or 'ambient music' radio station. Some people like white noise from a dedicated white noise generator, a CD or an FM radio tuned away from any station. Masking will work as effectively with low frequencies as with high, but be wary of two things: firstly, do not use excessive noise that might damage your hearing, and secondly, do not also mask important sounds like doorbells, alarms or the complaints of your family and co-workers.

Domestic low energy lighting has improved immensely since it was first available, and most of the branded compact fluorescent bulbs are quiet and flicker-free once they have warmed up. They can begin to exhibit some flicker and high-frequency hums as they age. Some of the latest LED lighting exhibits far worse flickering, although this might improve as the technology matures. Unfortunately, there is no escape from flickering, motion and brightly-coloured commotion outside the home, especially in shops and shopping centres. One of the most intense times of year for flickering and moving lights is in the run-up to Christmas when every kind of new and old flashing sign competes for attention. We are trying to say in this chapter that avoidance is not the best strategy for dealing with sensory issues, but in this instance it may be appropriate to practice moderation — be aware of the intensity of sensations and the effect that they are having on you, and be prepared to limit your exposure by choosing quieter places to shop or to spend less time shopping. If a decorated, flashing Christmas tree is difficult for you in a shared living area, then explaining which elements bother you will allow you to compromise on decorations that everybody, including you, find pleasing. This might be as simple as using continuous, non-flashing yellow lights (the old-fashioned kind) and putting all the flashing lights in a hallway or other area that everyone can enjoy, but do not bother you when you are trying to relax or work.

Touch (or tactile) sensations are often intense. People who feel intense, unpleasant skin sensations will often use techniques that are called tactile defensiveness to avoid those sensations — perhaps you keep your hands balled-up in a fist when you are out, or wear heavy, full-length clothing even when it is warm, or you have systematically cut the tags out of every item of clothing. You might also have a collection of clothing that looks great, but you never, ever wear — and you can't throw away the items that were expensive or were gifts! Perhaps you always feel that you have to 'rub out' any light touch. All of these are signs of tactile sensitivity. Natural fabrics (cotton, linen and wool) are generally more comfortable than synthetics. Full-length sleeves and trousers protect sensitive skin, but you may find that a number of thinner full-length layers are more socially acceptable than one thick layer — wearing a hooded fleece or winter coat might make it look like you are about to leave, or don't want to stay.

Food can be a real problem for some people. Eating is one of the few experiences where we engage all five senses (taste, smell, sight, hearing and texture) simultaneously, one of the other occasions being sex. Eating is therefore a very intense experience, and should be pleasurable. However the texture of food, its variety or its unfamiliarity can make some people gag, no matter how hard they try to eat what is on offer. Perhaps you are always eating the same limited diet of dishes, always cooked and served in exactly the same way. Perhaps you become inexplicably upset if the vegetables touch the meat, or if there is even the tiniest hint of herbs in the food. If you are preparing your own food and eating at home, then the main issue to be aware of is that your diet is healthy and balanced, and is not excessively fatty, sugary or salty. If you are not preparing your own meals, then perhaps you could begin to do so in order that you have more control over eating food that appeals to you. When eating food that others prepare and you don't enjoy, it may be easier to eat the unpleasant parts first or to interleave them with the enjoyable portions. Sometimes there may be a choice of texture — for instance the pink or the well-done parts of a roasted joint, or by mashing vegetables and adding gravy (or choosing not to have gravy, if you prefer drier food). Remember that food is a social activity and the social aspects of eating often exceed its nutritional value, so it is always important to be polite at shared mealtimes.

Smell is an area where most of us will meet a few individuals far more sensitive to certain odours than ourselves — odour, especially human or animal body odours, are a big social taboo. Despite odour being part of social and sexual bonding, humans spend immense amounts of time and money trying to eradicate, isolate and mask it with cleansers, air-conditioning and perfume.

Unfortunately (for us) the cure is often worse than the problem — the smell of human waste products is preferable to the same smell **and** an artificial pine-fresh air-spray. The most effective approach to dealing with unwanted smells at home is good airflow, frequent cleaning and laundering dirty clothes. (Of course minimising smell is going to be at odds with minimising sound, where you want to shut yourself in with lots of sound-absorbing materials). Using unscented soap, unscented clothes detergent and finding cosmetic and shaving products with the lowest levels of perfume can be hard, but is not impossible. Fabric softeners, toilet fresheners, floor and kitchen cleaning products and supposed air-fresheners are among the worst culprits. Burning a plain candle (in a safe candle holder) can help to eliminate some smells, including tobacco smoke and some solvents.

2.1.1 Learning to handle unpleasant sensations

Learning to handle unpleasant sensory experiences, whether noise, smell or any other, comes down to managing exposure, increasing personal tolerance of the experiences and having coping strategies for your own aversive reactions. The first issue — managing exposure — is something that you will never have complete personal control over, unless you wish to become a hermit. Some exposure is open to compromise with people you live, study or work with — for instance it may be reasonable to expect not to have to listen to loud music or power-tools at times when you should be studying or working. It should also be reasonable to ask that people do not eat food with strong smells (or that involve a lot of mouth noises, like crisps or bubble-gum) in a shared work space — and that they dispose of food waste in an appropriate place, like the kitchen or outside bins, rather than an office or bedroom waste paper basket.

However, not all unpleasant sensory exposure is ever going to be within your control if you wish to live a fulfilled and involved life. Some people will not understand your sensory issues, others will trivialise them and on many occasions the noise, flickering light and smell are an unavoidable consequence of everyday activities that people take for granted. Keeping sight of the benefits can often make the unpleasant much more bearable. Going to work, earning an income and having a relationship with colleagues is a huge incentive to put up with the sensory issues that almost any workplace involves.

An important part of managing exposure, when exposure can be moderated, is the ability to predict both what your own issues are and the activities that are your personal triggers. You might not even be aware of the precise sensory issues that you have because sensory exposure so often occurs as a collection of related experiences. Finger-food or buffets are often a feature of stand-up social occasions with a lot of strangers, brief conversations and dressing for show, including wearing perfume and after-shave. A roomful of these different exposures from so many people can leave you dazed and nauseous, without knowing which elements of the social occasion make you feel unwell and you might blame everything from the jumbled conversation to the rich food. I blamed my own food intolerance and nausea on buffet food for years until I realised that I was suffering from an excess of 'social calories', the sheer emotional effort of making and breaking social contact with so many people in a short space of time. The food itself, as I know now, is perfectly edible to me, as long as I limit the event to just showing my face and leaving as soon as it is polite to do so. An occupational therapist can be an excellent source of help in pinpointing your own specific sensory issues and separating the issues that cause the most personal distress from other sensory exposures that you usually feel with them.

Some methods of building tolerance include progressive exposure, a 'sensory diet' (often supervised by an occupational therapist) and sound therapy (auditory integration training). These methods have mixed results, and while some people report great success, others report no benefit whatsoever. We are not aware of any reports of having **worse** sensory issues after therapy, so they do not do any harm — except, of course, that private therapy can be very expensive and can run for many sessions.

Methods of improving your coping skills when you do experience unpleasant sensory situations include meditation or yoga, progressive muscular relaxation (PMR), mindfulness therapy and controlled breathing. All of these can be used 'in the moment' to cope with anxiety or rising panic that occurs during a stressful sensory experience, but all are very much more effective if they are practised regularly, preferably at times of peace and calm in a safe environment. The recall of the safe, peaceful environment helps during exposure to anxiety and chaos elsewhere. Meditation or yoga are taught in many health centres, in some schools and through GP or HSE services. There are many books on using yoga to achieve personal calm, and although some yoga books are associated with religious beliefs, it is unlikely to conflict with most people's religious (or even atheist) beliefs. Progressive muscular relaxation is a method of progressively tensing and then relaxing each set of muscles in your body, from toes to face, in time with slow breathing and thinking about a pleasant and safe place. Progressive muscular relaxation is an effective way of reaching a state of calm while retaining a sense of personal control, which can be recalled during times of stress. Progressive muscular relaxation is used within anxiety management courses and other therapies in the HSE and other health centres — there are very many CDs available in bookshops containing spoken instructions and mood music to listen to and practice PMR in your own bedroom or other safe place. Mindfulness is another form of meditative therapy that has come to the fore in recent years as an effective method of getting in touch with bodily sensations and emotional feelings, often using quiet and slow breathing to become aware of the immediate surroundings and then aware of the sensations within your body. Mindfulness is one of the most frequent techniques used within psychological therapy practised by the HSE, and there are many books in general bookshops explaining the techniques used. The last technique, and the most immediate, is something that can be practised in moments of stress as well as during calm — breathe in while slowly counting to, perhaps 5, and then out while slowly counting to 5. Repeat the cycle of in and out for ten breaths. The more often that you use a technique like this (there are many variants), the more effective the results will be.

Most of us are too old or too self-conscious to get away with carrying a Linus blanket or comforter, but there are plenty of adult alternatives that can provide a familiar, predictable sensory comforter. This might be an article of clothing like a scarf, but key-fobs or strings of beads (like a rosary) are very good sensory comforters that you can hold in your hand, in or out of your pocket, without attracting any attention — counting through beads, especially sets that have marker beads, can be combined with slow breathing.

2.2 Psychological and emotional issues

People who have difficulty understanding emotions, both their own emotions and other people's emotions, have one form of impaired empathy. This is called impaired cognitive empathy, or impaired theory of mind. The other form is impaired emotional empathy, an inability to feel your own or other people's emotions — and people with autism spectrum disorder certainly do **feel** emotions, even if those feelings are difficult to identify, name and respond to appropriately. One consequence of impaired cognitive empathy is that behaviour can seem inappropriate to other people, and we misunderstand social situations. These inappropriate behaviours can be interpreted, or misinterpreted, as a variety of psychological disorders that have entered popular vocabulary, such as being paranoid, having ADHD or OCD.

One consequence of not recognizing emotions is the inability to discern the intent of other people's actions, or guessing the wrong intention, or indeed wrongly guessing that there was an intention when there was none at all. An example is to assume that you were pushed on purpose when someone bumps into you by accident. Assuming intent, and assuming a bad intention, might be an evolutionary defensive reaction to try to keep us safe in the face of unknown threats, but is not appropriate to most situations in modern society. There is plenty of evidence that always assuming a suspicious reaction to unknown intent will not make you any better at judging risk, and it certainly limits opportunities. If you assume a bad intention every time someone bumps into you or speaks to you brusquely, then you will perceive the world to be more hostile than it really is, and this may decrease your social opportunities and your willingness to participate in social activities. This tendency to suspicion of intents can be interpreted as paranoia or even, when suspicions are expressed verbally, as psychotic. In a clinical setting (for instance if you have a psychiatric assessment, or are admitted to a psychiatric hospital for treatment), then frequent mistakes about other people's intentions can be mistaken for paranoid delusions that indicate psychosis or even schizophrenia. A prior diagnosis of an autism spectrum disorder will provide some protection against a mistaken diagnosis of psychosis. In a social setting, being called paranoid can create a strong sense of social exclusion and isolation.

ADHD, which stands for attention-deficit hyperactivity disorder, is a behavioural disorder in which a person is restless, easily distracted, gets bored without mental or physical stimulation and sometimes with 'bad' behaviour in settings like school classrooms. ADHD (or ADD) is actually quite common in combination with an autism spectrum disorder, but is not a core symptom. ADHD has come into common speech as meaning restless or easily bored and people even talk about "feeling a bit ADHD" when they are bored or not able to focus. Some of the symptoms of autism, including difficulties with understanding social communication, heightened hearing sensitivity or tactile defensiveness, are easily confused with either clinical or everyday ADHD. Understanding why you feel "a bit ADHD" on any particular day or in any particular setting can be a big help in dealing with the triggers that are distracting or the social issues that prevent you from engaging socially with individuals or groups.

OCD is often used colloquially to refer to any tendency towards tidiness or order that is more than other people. Even keeping books or a music collection in order might be called OCD. In a clinical setting, obsessive-compulsive disorders include behaviours where it feels necessary to repeat a non-functional routine until it has been performed a set number of times, or to some arbitrary level of correctness. It includes the repetition of functional routines (such as washing) long after the function has been achieved, as well as patterns of pervasive thoughts that will not go away (such as the 'chattering monkeys' when you rethink an event over and over). Clinical OCD refers to the **distressing** repetition of routines that may (such as excessive hand-washing) result in personal harm. The colloquial OCD that we often have is usually associated with pleasure or, at least, security. If you feel better for sharpening every pencil, even the already sharp pencils, before you start work, then that routine is probably a useful centering activity that provides personal comfort and prepares you for the task ahead, knowing that your tools are all ready. As long as the preparation routines have not replaced the activity, this is not a negative. If you want to catalogue every song in your music collection and keep the discs in order, then you are sure to avoid being upset because you avoid losing track of items you love. Other people (including parents and medical professionals) may see some of your routines as non-functional, repetitive behaviours that tend towards OCD — but if you are not distressed by a compulsion outside your control, then you can view these behaviours as increasing the predictability and security of the world around you.

One consequence of being noticed as different, and of the various labels like having special needs, or being paranoid, ADHD or OCD is that people can bully or exclude you from social groups. These problems tend to worsen as pupils progress from primary into secondary school, and then decrease in third level education or employment. Although less frequent, bullying does exist in higher education and the workplace, and it can be far more subtle and far more destructive than crude group bullying that occurs in the playground. Most schools, colleges and workplaces have a policy on bullying and harassment, often called a dignity policy (it is a legal requirement to have a policy). Organisations differ greatly in recognizing and acting on bullying, and in some environments it is endemic and widely tolerated as 'part of growing up'. If you have difficulty understanding the intentions of others, difficulty recognizing distinct emotions and do not easily fit into social groups, then you might not be able to accurately distinguish bullying. It is very important to discuss social difficulties or your unhappiness with other people — parents, siblings, a student counsellor or a workplace human resources employee — especially when you do not understand other people's behaviour towards you. Correctly identifying and naming bullying behaviour is often all it takes to stop bullying, as long as your peers and people in charge are willing to identify bullying behaviours for what they are.

2.2.1 Anxiety and depression

The effects of social impairment, emotional processing and sensory reactions — always being on edge and rarely relaxing or feeling safe — have a lifelong impact on psychological well-being. The most immediate effect is anxiety, which can manifest as social anxiety, generalised anxiety disorder or panic attacks. One of the long-term effects of heightened anxiety is an increased risk of depression.

Anxiety is treatable, with varying degrees of success, using first line treatments of 'talking therapies' and physical activity or exercise. The second line treatment with prescription drugs. Talking therapies include cognitive-behavioural therapy (CBT, the currently most favoured psychological therapy), dialectic behaviour therapy (DBT), psychodynamic psychotherapy and other forms of verbal support and counselling. Talking therapies are preferred over the quick fix of medication because of the long history of drug dependency and over-use from miracle drugs like Valium (benzodiazepine), an extremely effective anxiety treatment developed in the 1960s and widely over-prescribed ever since. Anxiety medication remains an extremely effective option, and ad libitum (when needed) use of small doses can help deal with immediate incidents of anxiety, particularly predictable events like air flights, job interviews or weddings. Sustained or excessive use diminishes the drugs' effectiveness, builds tolerance to its beneficial effects and risks dependency (addiction).

Depression is a sustained low mood accompanied by feelings of worthlessness, guilt, loss of interest in activities that used to be pleasurable, fatigue and possibly thoughts that life is not worth continuing. Depression can be a natural reaction to traumatic life events such as bereavement or unemployment, or it can continue to become a mood disorder that limits any kind of normal functioning. The first line of treatment is again talking therapies, but antidepressant drugs are more often prescribed, and are prescribed early, alongside talking therapy. Treatment for depression is the same for everyone, whether autistic or not, with the advice that people with autism spectrum disorder may be more susceptible to the effects of psycho-active drugs than other people. As a result, antidepressants may be effective at a lower dose than many psychiatrists might expect. The psychiatric profession is obsessed with the latest, most technological advanced and most expensive drug therapies, despite having no clear understanding of what causes depression or how the drugs function. There is no clear evidence that modern drugs are any more effective than earlier generations of antidepressants, although there is generally less risk of accidental or deliberate overdose. Some of the oldest drugs, such as sertraline and tricyclic antidepressants have been found to be particularly effective in treating depression in people with autism spectrum disorder.

Physical activity and a balanced diet (including eating any form of breakfast every day) are consistently linked with increased self-esteem and mental well-being. These interventions are low-cost and entirely within your own control.

Running, brisk walking or an exercise regimen like 5BX can be done with minimal change to your daily routine, and everyone is recommended to take some moderate to vigorous exercise on at least 5 days each week.

2.2.2 Meltdowns (and tantrums)

What is the difference between a meltdown and a tantrum? Many people observing one or the other will be quite unable to tell the difference, unless it is explained to them, yet the wrong response can make a manageable situation into an extremely unpleasant situation that might be avoided. Put simply, a tantrum is an emotional reaction to real or perceived injustice that is directed towards the goal of righting the wrong. A meltdown is a response to sensory overload, without any goal. Both can be upsetting or frightening for an observer, especially a loved one.

The toddler wanting a sweet is the stereotype of a tantrum, and it describes explosive outbursts of rage in adults just as well as children who throw themselves screaming on a supermarket floor. There is a real or imagined unfair situation and shouting, screaming and throwing things is intended to get your own way, often when all attempts are politeness and reason have failed. People with language difficulties and people who have problems interpreting other people's emotions — that includes some people with autism spectrum disorders — are going to experience real or perceived injustice more often than people who do not, and tantrums are common in children with autism. A tantrum will stop immediately the goal (getting the sweet, or your own way) has been achieved or the unreasonableness of the complaint has been understood. If the parent does not give in and the child does not see reason, then tantrums can escalate until a child is at risk of harming someone, usually him or herself. Unmanaged anger in adolescents is more dangerous than in toddlers because they are physically larger and capable of using objects as make-do weapons — throwing plates or tools, for instance, can cause serious harm. If you experience outbursts of anger that you are not able to manage, then you can practice some of the self-soothing and calming techniques we describe in this chapter and you can seek professional help through an anger-management course. Anger-management is widely recognised as a serious problem that people who experience anger need help from professionals in bringing under control, because unmanaged anger is a risk to themselves and to people they share space with. You can ask for referral to an anger management course through your school, GP or any health professional that you feel able to talk to about the issue. Understanding that you have an issue with anger-management and dealing with injustice — whether real or imagined injustice — may be enough to discuss it with the people you live with or have problems with. If other people understand the stresses that you feel and the difficulty you have expressing a sense of grievance, then they will be prepared to spend longer listening to you and trying harder to understand your perspective, averting the outbursts. An adult tantrum can be frightening to watch and you might avoid discussing it because the event is so embarrassing to live down, but it is all the more important to understand and explain it.

Meltdowns are more specific to people with autism spectrum disorder, particularly people who have sensory issues or difficulty understanding their own emotions. An extreme meltdown might be triggered by the sounds of a shopping centre, the crush of all the other people shopping, the difficulty finding some particular item that has been moved when the shop was last rearranged, topped off by your parent or partner asking you to hurry up and make your mind up. The explosion of senses and unidentifiable emotions seems to create an electrical storm inside your head — some people report noises like static and flashes of light behind their eyes — and an extreme urge to run away and hide somewhere dark, quiet and safe. Instead of calm, the noise just gets louder and more insistent, the pushing feels like being punched and then you have no idea what you are saying — it means "please be quiet and let me get calm", but those are definitely not the words that come out, if anything intelligible comes out at all. Not every body becomes excitable and uncontrolled at this point, and some people will simply become stiff and unresponsive, although both responses are escapes from the unpleasant sensations inside and outside their bodies. The animated and excitable meltdown might involve shouting, a dictionary of inappropriate (or even well-chosen) swear words, pushing or hitting and can result in security guards, Gardai or an ambulance being called if it causes disruption in a public place. If a meltdown is treated like a tantrum — trying to right the injustice or to reason with the person who is melting down — it will only add to the sensory overload and make things worse. An aggressive response from security guards or paramedics will also make things worse. The only way out of a meltdown is to remove the sensory overload, to provide space and to make the time for the person to recover some calm. In a public place or in a setting with strangers, it can be helpful to explain that the person is not drunk or on drugs and that he or she has a specific sensory disability that requires some space and calm. Some charities — the National Autistic Society in the UK and Irish Autism Action are two — have autism alert cards that explain some of these issues for security and medical staff. Just having the alert card in a wallet can provide some peace of mind if a public meltdown is an issue that worries you, even if you never have reason to show it. I have occasionally been in situations in hospitals and airports where I have been subjected to intimate examinations that I responded to so badly that security guards were called to calm me, which made things much worse, and have started carrying one of these cards to present if I feel things are getting difficult for me to manage.

As with the sensory issues mentioned above, prediction and moderation are really important in managing situations that lead to meltdowns. If you are lucky enough to be able to feel the triggers for your own meltdown situations, then you may be able to slow down, back away from the situation and avoid the meltdown completely. If you are with other people and can explain that you are not going to be able to cope, then they can help you find a safer, quieter space to gather your thoughts and establish some inner calm. This can mean a break to take a coffee or snack, or it might mean going home and finishing the shopping or outing on another day. If your are unlucky, then the sensations that should be acting as warnings that your trigger factors are being tripped will also be signals to your conscious mind that you need to get a move on with the very thing that is causing the build-up to a meltdown — a bit like accelerating when you see that your car is almost out of petrol. Every effort that you spend on trying to do things faster, more intensely or more efficiently will only bring you to meltdown that much sooner, and probably more violently. Having people around you who recognize your responses can help if they can recognize the early signs of impending meltdown and help you to slow down. Some of the relaxation techniques described in this chapter — particularly mindfulness or meditation techniques — can help you to learn what your bodily sensations mean and to learn to recognize when to take things slower, or simply stop what you are doing and take time out to rest.

In a workplace setting you can discuss issues like this with an occupational health officer or human resources manager, and find techniques like 'power napping' or a quiet room to allow you to centre yourself when you feel that you are experiencing sensory or emotional overload.

2.2.3 Aggression and self-harm

Sometimes emotional distress can become so difficult to deal with that people choose to inflict injuries on themselves, often by cutting with a sharp object, burning their skin or hitting a hard surface with a fist or head. These forms of *self-harm* can act as a release in the immediate term, but if you are using them (or thinking of using them) it is a big warning sign that you are not coping with your emotions. The same applies if you occasionally or regularly lose your temper violently, especially if any of this behaviour either frightens or endangers you or other people. For long-term psychological well-being, it is essential to seek help with the emotional issues that underlie any form of aggressive or self-harmful behaviours. A good place to start, especially if you have trouble identifying or explaining your distressing emotions, is with the plain facts of what kind of behaviour you use or are thinking about.

2.3 Asperger syndrome and health issues

Some day-to-day issues involve intimate questions or intimate examinations, which can be both embarrassing and distressing — especially when there is a lot of sensory or emotional feelings. Sometimes it can help to tell people that you have an autism spectrum disorder (or carry some form of autism information card explaining it). If you have difficulty identifying and talking about emotions then it can help to say so. We discuss the specific issues of communicating ill-health and communicating emotional difficulties in Chapter 7.

2.4 Medicines and other drugs

It can safely be said that there are no drugs (nor any diets or other medical interventions) that treat the core symptoms of autism. Neither is autism 'curable', by any form of therapy. The proven therapies for the core symptoms of autism are entirely behavioural and social interventions that help people to discover their own emotions, to learn social skills and to adapt their behaviours when they are inappropriate. It is not possible to avoid the debate over whether autism **should** be cured, if and when a cure is available, or if people with autism spectrum disorder are part of a natural continuum of humanity that should be left alone as natural variation. Our opinion is that the symptoms of autism cause discomfort, distress and misery in varying degrees to different people with autism, and to people who love and care for them. Just as with any other human condition that upsets physical or emotional well-being, we advocate therapies that help people to lead a satisfied and fulfilled life. We do not advocate 'normalising' people with autism, that is to say any form of 'cure' which has the primary purpose of making autistic symptoms invisible or training people with autism to 'act normal' for the sake of not standing out.

As a reader of this book you will probably feel that you are too old to benefit from any form of behavioural therapy or social training, but you would be quite wrong. It is true that behavioural and social programmes are far more effective when delivered as early as possible, and that the benefits diminish with increasing age, but there is no such thing as too old. If you have never had the benefit of an occupational therapist assessment, you will undoubtedly benefit from a professional assessment that might uncover sensory and behavioural issues that you never knew you had, or for which you have learned very effective masking behaviours — some of which would possibly benefit from therapy and some of which may actually be negative, aversive masking behaviours that limit opportunity. An obvious one is not going out and limiting social contact because friendships cause pain. Your aversive behaviour certainly avoids the immediate negative pain, but there is no positive benefit either. Social skills can be learned at any age.

At the time of writing there is no national programme to provide any form of adult (18 and over) therapy to people with autism spectrum disorder, although a bill has recently been introduced to the Dáil to provide for a national autism strategy that would include adult outreach services. There are regional supports in some areas through charities, listed in the back of this book. There is also support from psychiatric outpatient services of the HSE, if you also have or have had in the past a diagnosis of a psychiatric disorder, most commonly anxiety or depression. There may also be support where any of the symptoms of autism are sufficiently limiting that they are recognized as a disability that limits occupational or social opportunities, particularly if you also had a statement of special educational need while in school and have continued contact with the HSE.

2.4.1 Prescription drugs and over-the-counter medicine

As stated above, there are no cures for autism and no prescription drugs for the core symptoms of autism. There are many drugs used to help with symptoms and to help with the side-effects of living with autism. These drugs are mostly classed as psychiatric drugs and are prescribed to treat side-effects of living with autism that would be classed as psychiatric illness if they existed in isolation. The most frequently prescribed classes of drugs are anxiolytics (anti-anxiety medication), stimulants that aid concentration and anti-psychotics that help deal with aggression and pervasive negative thoughts. Many people with autism spectrum disorder, including the author and animal-handling expert Temple Grandin, state that drugs can be effective at far lower doses than those normally prescribed and that psychiatric medication should start at a lower dose and be ramped up more slowly in people with autism.

Anti-anxiety drugs deal with stress and anxiety through many different (and often unknown) mechanisms. Some of the drugs that are prescribed for lifelong anxiety, generalized anxiety disorder and social anxiety were originally developed for other purposes, as antidepressants, anti-epileptics and circulatory drugs (for instance beta-blockers). Their side-effects in reducing anxiety were happy accidents discovered during clinical trials for their original purpose or during long-term use. The frontline wonder-drugs of the 1950s and 1960s were benzodiazepines and their relatives, the most famous of which is Valium, but these drugs act fairly quickly, have a short half-life before being metabolised and excreted, and are tolerated gradually over time leading to the need to increase doses as they become less effective, which risks long-term problems of dependency and addiction. Other drugs such beta-blockers, buspirone or the anti-convulsant pregabalin (Lyrica) have a longer half-life, act more slowly and do not result in long-term tolerance and dependency. However, some people with autism have used small doses of ad libitum (i.e. as and when needed) benzodiazepines for the long-term management of anxiety very effectively, without obvious dependency and without requesting rising doses.

Stimulants such as ritalin are one of the most commonly prescribed medications for treating attention-deficit disorder (ADD) and attention-deficit hyperactivity disorder (ADHD). They assist mental focus and can help people to ignore distractions. Somebody who is easily distracted and has difficulty focusing may benefit from the use of a stimulant. An effective treatment for anxiety may have the same, or better, outcome benefits in managing focus and distraction.

Anti-psychotic medications have a range of effects on thinking and behaviour that can be useful in managing autism — useful either to the person with autism or people caring for them. Anti-psychotics can be very effective at reducing the negative effects of pervasive negative thoughts, the kind of unwelcome and unpleasant thoughts that are associated with obsessive-compulsive disorder (OCD) and which do not respond to any amount of reasoned thinking. Cognitive-behavioural therapy is the recommended first line of therapy for pervasive negative thinking, but drugs can be helpful when thoughts are particularly invasive, particularly limiting of normal function or include aggressive or self-harmful thoughts, including suicidal thoughts. Anti-psychotics also have a rapid calming effect on agitation, aggression and violence. If you have uncontrollable agitation or aggression, then you may have benefit from anti-psychotics when no other calming therapies are effective — with a downside that the side-effects include a mental fog, drowsiness and inability to concentrate, throughout the entire day following a dose of anti-psychotic. There is also a danger that anti-psychotics are used by carers to make patients more manageable in care settings, even when their levels of agitation or aggression are an entirely natural response to the degree of boredom or social exclusion that they are experiencing in care. This use of over-medication to control difficult behaviour has been termed a 'chemical cosh', the pharmaceutical equivalent of being hit over the head to induce calm. A triple-whammy consisting of an antipsychotic, a sleeping medication and the allergy drug anti-histamine (which causes drowsiness and also has a synergistic effect making the first two more potent) is frequently used in psychiatric care and can be prescribed in a home setting. Such use is for the benefit of carers and not for the benefit of the patient (except in reducing self-harm and conflict such as physical restraint). However, do consider that anti-psychotic drugs can be effective in dealing with persistent and disturbing thoughts, especially in low doses and under your own control — although obtaining a low-dose, ad libitum prescription may be difficult without a lot of explanation or an understanding psychiatrist.

Self-medication includes any variety of medication using over-the-counter (OTC) products that are not prescribed, whether pepper-mint oil for abdominal cramps or chondroitin for joint health. Food supplements (vitamins and minerals) are the most common form of self-medication product. Supplements have been reported to be beneficial by many people with ASD and their parents. Supplements can be expensive. Scientific evidence of the value of food supplementation is inconclusive (this applies in general, and not only specifically to people with ASD) and it is a recognized problem that funding and disciplinary interests are not aligned with health objectives — minerals and vitamins can not generate the same profit as patented drugs. Specific supplements that some people recommend in ASD are magnesium (liquid essence), omega-3 and omega-6 fatty acids, vitamin B (B-complex, B-6, B-12), copolymer Q-10, vitamins A, C & E (the antioxidants) and probiotics (including probiotic yoghurt). You can find a lot of books at shelf-mark 613.2 in your local library and in books like "Nutrition for Dummies" by Carol Ann Rinzler — there is no mystery about diet and nutrition, for someone with autism as for any other person. Surprisingly little peer-reviewed research has been conducted on the impact of diet and nutrition on people with autism spectrum disorder. The majority of studies that have been conducted have been too small to detect any benefit, but we equally do not know if there is no benefit. Some anecdotal reports, studies on laboratory animals and experiments in petri-dishes are improperly used to support unproven theories about autism diets and cures. The worst examples (including some diets and remedies sold over the internet) are exploitative or even harmful.

Most people in Ireland eat too much and have an unbalanced diet and people with autism have more restricted diets than many other people. People with autism may have a less effective metabolism and more gastro-intestinal or abdominal symptoms — whether that is true or not, a healthy, balanced diet aids physical and mental health. Eating five portions of fresh fruit and vegetables every day, reducing excess calories from fat and carbohydrates, and reducing known irritants (alcohol, caffeine and chocolate) are all beneficial. A healthy, balanced diet is a necessary starting point before using dietary supplements or any investigation of an individual or exclusion diet.

Some people with autism feel better on exclusionary diets and some parents report that their children's behaviour improves on exclusionary diets — diet is one of the most frequent interventions and is used by the majority of parents of children with autism. Starting from a balanced healthy diet, exclusions should be assessed by a gastro-entological review of the individual's intolerance to specific foods, such as casein or gluten. "Feeling better" or "behaving better" are subjective judgements that should be treated with care, especially when those judgements are made by parents imposing an exclusionary diet on their children. An exclusionary diet can be expensive and time-intensive, as well as increasing social isolation — GFCF birthday cakes, children's food and restaurant food are a rarity. A number of organisations and alternative therapists promote testing for toxins and food intolerances using techniques that are not scientifically proven. There are advertisements for tests for heavy metals, environmental toxins, yeast and bacterial infections, nutritional deficiencies, food intolerance — the same organisation often also sells therapeutic diet guides and supplements for people who test positive for these factors. Some of these interventions may be beneficial (although the evidence is anecdotal), most do no harm, and some are harmful. Dietary interventions provide people with a level of personal control that can improve quality of life, irrespective of any nutritional benefit. There is no doubt that some individuals have severe food intolerances (e.g. coeliacs), but food intolerance should be tested by a gastroenterologist. Appropriate exclusions hugely improve the quality of life of food-intolerant individuals.

2.4.2 Other drugs (both legal and illegal)

As with prescription drugs, there are claims that people with autism spectrum disorder are affected more by mood-altering and psycho-active products than others, and therefore more affected by widely available legal and illegal drugs. People with autism are more vulnerable to some of the dangers associated with drug use, including peer-pressure to take drugs to fit in and the dangers associated with being alone during overdose (which includes excessive alcohol consumption). Social isolation or social exclusion during or after taking drugs to excess vastly increases the dangers of overdose.

Alcohol and caffeine are probably the most common forms of off-label self-medication. As with other drugs, people use and abuse them because the effects feel good (at least initially) and because they are associated with enhancing some forms of performance. Taking caffeine can stimulant mental and physical function and is widely used in coffee, cola drinks, tea and the 'energy drinks' that contain combinations of caffeine, guarana and taurine in varying combinations. An occasional coffee can stimulate mental performance and help late-night study before an exam. Surviving on high-caffeine drinks can cause abdominal irritation, disturbed sleep and paranoia at its most extreme. Alcohol is a nervous system depressant which has an immediate, pleasant calming effect for most people who use it. If only we could stop at this point, it might have more benefit than most people experience, but a lot of people continue until alcohol affects their judgement, limits physical performance (such as driving ability) and reduces social inhibitions to often dangerous levels. Alcohol is responsible for more violent disorder, more hospital admissions and more lifelong ill-health than any other drug abuse. However, that initial calming effect and its associated lowering of inhibition (or social anxiety) is so effective for most people that alcohol is associated with almost all forms of social gathering at every socio-economic level of society. Many people with autism spectrum disorder feel that they are able to overcome their nerves and fit in better with a few drinks.

Street drugs that are easily available in Ireland include the prescription anti-anxiety benzodiazepines, cannabis (resin / hash, herbal marijuana and oil / black), cocaine, crystal meth, the party drug ecstasy, heroin, the veterinary anaesthetic ketamine, liberty cap (psilocybin) mushrooms, LSD (acid), the depressant methadone used for heroin treatment, solvents, the stimulant speed (amphetamine) and steroids (anabolic and androgenic drugs). Drugs can provide immediate euphoric effects, a sense of confidence, detachment from reality and intense, dreamlike states of consciousness that are plainly enjoyable and desirable to people who use drugs — that is why illegal drugs are so widely distributed and so widely consumed despite significant criminal penalties. The illegal drug ecstasy (which should be MDMA, but is often adulterated or diluted in street pills) has been taken in greater volume than almost any prescribed pharmaceutical drug, with fewer instances of death or illness than caused by aspirin. A major health problem of ecstasy (and all illegal drugs) is accidental contamination or deliberate adulteration with substitutes that can be far more dangerous than the original MDMA. Despite the widespread publicity of the dangers of street drugs, the legal drugs alcohol and tobacco are responsible for far more social disturbance, domestic violence and ill-health than illegal drugs.

In addition to the classified street drugs, there is a continuously changing market in mood-altering drugs sold through headshops and other channels that attempt to evade legal penalties through loopholes and sheer novelty — a drug can not be illegal until it has been classified. Some of these products are industrial chemicals or natural products with intense (and under-studied) effects, some are actually street or prescription drugs in disguise and some are simply scams without any significant effects. Some of the products are sold under euphemisms such as 'bath-salts', which are substituted cathinones having a stimulant effect similar to that of cocaine or amphetamines. These products deliberately skirt the boundaries of illegality and are the source of a disproportionate number of hospital admissions and other ill-effects because their contents and effects are unregulated and unpredictable — added to which, the precise effect on any individual is an additional unknown.

One issue that has been raised with some street drugs is the possibility that mood-altering effects can overcome social impairments or other symptoms associated with autism, much as the claimed effect of alcohol in helping people overcome nerves. Both cannabis and ketamine are the subject of formal academic trials on their effects in rats and even people with autism spectrum disorder. The compounds used in academic experiments are pure and of tightly controlled doses of selective active compounds. The outcomes do not at present show sufficient promise to extend limited laboratory experiments into clinical trials.

3 Relationships *(Diarmuid Heffernan)*

3.1 Relating to strangers and less familiar people

The process of inter-relationships between humans is a complex and evolving one. As a species we have spent millennia trying to develop and explore the basis for different facets of human interaction and we are still in the process of discovering new ways in which we relate to each other and why. One of the most interesting issues of the moment is the interaction between technology and humanity. Many now feel for example that technology has passed out humanity in the sense that human beings no longer understand the effect technology is having on human development, particularly children. The pace at which the world is changing is outpacing the rigours of research in that scientific research takes a considerable amount of time to become accepted as scientific fact and by the time this process is complete the research is potentially obsolete as the world has moved beyond it. What this all means for you is that the world of social relations is complex and ever changing, however there are some ways in which you can make interactions with others easier on yourself. One such way is by trying to look at the social world from the point of view of those not on the autism spectrum. So for example you may find yourself at a bus stop on a rainy day with a stranger who says to you 'what a terribly wet day'. Now you may think to yourself that is an exercise in stating the obvious on their part but in reality it is a little more complex than that. When the person is saying this, or indeed in any other situation where there is 'small talk', it is an expression of acknowledgement, that is to say that the person is acknowledging you there (this is across the species, for example dogs sniff each other, or bark at each other). It is a very simple way of communicating with you. So rather than thinking of the words as being superfluous, try to see that the person may in fact be just trying to be friendly, maybe they are lonely, maybe they think you look friendly or that you remind them of someone! Ultimately, small talk is an integral part of the way many people use language in an everyday setting, and language is a vital aspect in providing the social glue which binds societies together. You may rather talk about something more meaningful to you but other people may not ascribe the same meaning to a given subject in the way that you do. It is best to try and stick to some simple rules when interacting with people in public spaces: be polite, be mannerly, try to accept that others may be trying to interact with you in a way that does not necessarily suit you or that you don't understand very well but for the most part people's motives are friendly. If you feel they are not being friendly then its best to politely remove yourself from the situation.

3.2 Shopping and other chores in public spaces

Going out alone to the shop or to run other errands in public spaces can cause anxiety, it can also be intimidating, frightening or even overwhelming at times but try not to let that stop you doing it! The fact is that the less you do of this, the harder it becomes, and despite the fact that each occasion may be very challenging, the less consistently you do it the more difficult each occasion will be. There are ways of making it easier for yourself. For example if you are grocery shopping, pick a time when you know it will be less busy, maybe during the day if it is possible or possibly later at night as there are many shops and convenience stores which are twenty four hour. If shopping in a convenience shop do bear in mind the potential cost implications as these shops tend to be more expensive than supermarkets. It may be worth going on quiet days or nights such as on Monday or Tuesday rather than the weekend — if that is possible. Also take the structure and layout of the shop into consideration. So a badly laid out shop in the busiest street in your town or city may be a recipe for anxiety and intimidation. You may never actually enjoy going to the shop but with time and practice and consideration to the above advice, it may become routine for you. If it is possible to go to the same shop at the same time it may be possible to make the experience less stressful as it becomes a routine. A further appendix to this is to have a shopping list. A shopping list will focus you on what you need to get and it speeds up the process.

Try not to get overly hung up on getting everything on the list if something is out of stock or not currently being sold in that shop (supermarket). Move on to your next item and you can figure out what to get instead as you move around the shop or when you get home. Take into consideration whether you would prefer to interact with the cashiers or not, if not, you may want to go to a shop which has self service tills, if you do then pick a shop where you are relatively comfortable interacting with the cashiers.

Going into public spaces in general may bring different types of challenges. Some may involve your interactions with others as discussed above, and others may have to do with the environment and the potential sensory issues inherent in particular spaces. There may be certain noises or smells which create sensory difficulties for you. There may also be visual stimuli which create difficulties for you, such as fluorescent lighting. It is again worth exploring which shops or supermarkets cause you the least amount of stress and anxiety, this may involve trial and error and it is important to persist even when you feel things have not gone as well as planned.

The built environment may also bring sensory difficulties, for example certain streets may be narrower and busier than others and so may force you to be in closer proximity to other people, or people may brush against you in a way that makes you feel uncomfortable. Again it may be worth looking into alternative times or days on these streets when they may be less busy. A further consideration for both shops/supermarkets and streets is having an 'escape route' for yourself — that is to say that you do not feel hemmed in and if you start to feel overwhelmed that there is a clear route out of the building or away from the street. If this happens you may want to find a way of calming yourself. You could do this by listening to calming music or your own voice (or someone who you find calms you) in a recorded refrain — reassuring yourself. A useful tip for many is to find an art gallery or library as these spaces are usually quiet and calm — and therefore potentially calming.

3.3 Recognizing friendship and hostility

As mentioned previously most people are well meaning and are not devious or hostile. This is not to say that all are well meaning however and it is important that you recognize hostility or even danger. In general terms cities and towns are at their most dangerous on weekend nights where there is alcohol involved, for example many pubs and clubs have smoking areas or have people congregating outside especially at weekends. You have a right to be on the street just the same as everyone else is but it is better to avoid dark or unlit streets or not to walk through congregated gangs of people. Also it is best to avoid verbal interaction with those who may be verbally aggressive or abusive towards you, it is best to ignore this and move away.

On a one-to-one basis you may feel that people you interact with such as a bus driver or shopkeeper are being hostile or unfriendly only to you while being friendly to others. If this is the case it may be, for example, because they are having a bad day or week. We cannot assume to know the reasons why someone is unfriendly in a shop or on a bus but we should not always assume it is because of something we have or have not done. It is also worth thinking about how much of your difficulty with others is down to previous negative experiences you may have had. It is therefore worth looking at how much of your negative social experience is observable, objective reality and how much arises from a sense of social exclusion. As we suggested above being polite and friendly is the most appropriate response, while taking into consideration we all have bad days! On the other hand people being unnecessarily brusque or rude is not something you should feel like you have to put up with and being assertive is also important. This means being verbally polite but firm on your rights and entitlements, it does not mean being argumentative, or aggressive. This is a delicate balancing act that no-one gets right all the time. Do not become disheartened however and do not let one incident affect the rest of your day or dictate your future ability to be assertive, it is best to let these feelings go and move on. As with most things in life we learn experientially and trial and error is intrinsic to the process.

The same principles may be applied to friendships. It is a trial and error process in recognizing and indeed maintaining friendships. There are no hard and fast rules or indeed definitive handbooks on friendship (although we include a guide to relationships in the resources section of this book), it is something which usually grows organically. There are some criteria for what constitutes a friendship however. So maybe in beginning to define what a friendship might be, we should look at what it is not. The person who talks to you at the bus stop is not a friend, but rather a friendly stranger. When people talk to you casually, but you do not spend any time in their company by design rather than accident or coincidence then that is not a friendship. A friendship should involve voluntarily spending time in each other's company, or have some things in common which you both enjoy doing or talking about together. Being acquainted with someone may just be knowing someone casually but without spending any time with them.

If you are lucky enough to have a friend or friends (most people crave friendship of one sort or another). It is vital that you try and nurture and maintain that friendship. So for example for most people friendship has to constitute a two way relationship where both parties have a mutual commitment to the friendship, therefore it would generally be expected that you would make an effort to contact or see the person as well as them contacting you. Friendship should have a reciprocal element to it because if there is only one party making the effort then it is not truly a friendship. Knowing what friends expect of you can be tricky and if someone is already a friend or could become a friend then honesty is the best policy in terms of discussing what you find difficult. For example, if you find meeting in a very crowded place stressful then its best to say this to your friend rather than avoid meeting them. If they are truly a friend then they will understand and agree to meet somewhere mutually enjoyable. Another vital component in maintaining a friendship is being there for the person and by this we mean being able to listen to their issues or news. It may also involve taking the initiative with your friendship. This may involve, for example, taking the person for a drink or a coffee (or inviting them to your abode for same if you do not want to talk about sensitive issues in a public space). It also helps to be aware that most people appreciate cards for Christmas, birthdays, anniversaries etc. If you have trouble remembering dates (as I do!) it helps to have them in a diary or on your phone as a reminder. A card with a nice message is generally fine.

In terms of remembering dates of birthdays, who to contact and when, and how frequently we propose devising an adaptation of the Leitner cards used for learning new languages. This method when adapted would use a version of the Leitner flash card techniques for relationships in that each relationship has a duration (e.g a week, month or year) and a card is moved to the back at each contact, the card at the front would require a call, e-mail or meeting.

3.4 Building social awareness

Building social awareness takes time. As mentioned earlier, social interaction and communication with others is a complex arena and no one gets it right all the time. The best way to learn is to learn experientially and this is sometimes a painful experience. Do not give up, however, as the rewards for learning from your experiences is an improved ability to read social situations and to read others. One important aspect of building social awareness is learning to read the intricacies of social language. For example many people may talk about a topic or even a person in an implied way without making direct reference to the person or subject in question. This may make it very difficult to interact with this type of conversation as you may be thinking to yourself — why don't they just say what they need to say directly! This is an area of your life that you will come to manage better through experience. The 'implied' conversation takes time to get used to (if you ever do) and you may always feel that being more direct is better. However it is very important to note that being too direct and/or honest can also create difficulties for you. For instance telling people who you don't know very well about your sex life might cause an embarrassed reaction in others. It is best to keep intimate details about yourself or spouse/partners/family between you and the parties concerned unless it is with trusted friends, family or appropriate professionals. One of the reasons for this is to protect yourself and those closest to you who may not want personal information related to them discussed in public. In a worst case scenario personal information about yourself given to someone who does not have your best interests at heart may be used to bully you or ridicule you. This is also true on the internet through blogs etc, and not just in face-to-face encounters.

It is also worth noting that most people use conversation to protect themselves. What we mean by this is that most people feel more comfortable verbally expressing safe topics while keeping their innermost feelings or thoughts to themselves as a way of protecting themselves, as exposing these thoughts or feelings may make them feel more vulnerable. This is essentially a layer, an extra coat of protection from the potential slings and arrows of the social world. What this also means is that people may say one thing but be feeling something different. So take a situation where a friend has had an argument with their partner about something very intimate. You may meet them and feel that they look sad, angry or upset but when you ask them how they are they say they are fine. In this situation it is likely they are not intentionally setting out to lie to you but they don't feel ready or able to talk to you about it in this moment. Despite the fact that now may always feel like the right time to discuss or analyse feelings etc or to understand a problem, it is best to respect people's wishes around this and allow them to deal with what they need to deal with in their own way and in their own time. 'Time heals' may not work for many people with AS but it is worth remembering that it does for many others.

3.5 Dating and being in a couple

Finding a partner in life is not easy, especially in a world that is so fast moving and atomised. There are very many single people as a result of the pace and structure of modern life. Many people feel that the best way of meeting someone is in social situations like in pubs or clubs. Generally these environments revolve around the imbibing of alcohol which diminishes people's inhibitions. If you like these environments and you find using alcohol (sensibly) allows you to be more relaxed and less anxious then you may find you can practice talking to members of the opposite sex. This is a learnt skill and again is only developed through trial and error. Some general points to remember are that it is unlikely that a man/woman that you meet in a pub or club is immediately going to share your enthusiasm for machine guns or indeed weapons of any kind! This is not to say that you should not have particular interests or hobbies that may be unique to you, but rather you don't talk about them immediately in this social arena. What might be more successful is asking the person what they are interested in and having a conversation about that. Bear in mind that the conversation will most likely be of the 'small talk' variety and the rules around not divulging very personal things about yourself still apply. If you feel the conversation is going well and there is reciprocation then you could ask for the person's number with a view to going on a date. Conversely if someone has approached you to talk to you they might ask you out on a date. Never feel pressurised into doing this, if you like them — then you may agree and if you are not sure — then you can always take their number and say you will think about it. It is not a binding agreement and people may (and do) change their minds.

Many people would rather not meet potential partners in pubs/clubs, but rather in spaces where alcohol is not a factor. There are increasing opportunities to meet others in different spaces now, such as through the internet. If you decide you would like to meet someone through the internet then it is advisable that you use a reputable internet dating site which is regulated and includes profiles of the person you may wish to go on a date with. There are other methods of meeting like-minded people, for example, some AS websites. You may also meet people with shared interests at night classes, meditation classes, yoga, martial arts etc.

Dating has some rigour attached to it which may or may not suit you, but it is best to be aware of. If you have asked someone on a date then be prepared to compromise on location especially if the other person has a distance to travel for the date. Going to the cinema is often a good first date as you can watch a movie then discuss it afterwards, so you immediately have a topic of conversation in common. If you agree to meet in a restaurant then we have some simple advice, do not assume the other person should or will pay, do not eat from the other person's plate! and try to engage the person in conversation about themselves (take note that this does not mean a form of inquisition or indeed that you produce a list of prepared questions — it is a date not an investigation!). Dating is also a matter of trial and error so be patient and be prepared to meet more than one person if your first date does not work out.

If you have met someone who is now a partner or spouse then you may be relieved to be done with the dating scene. You do however need to be conscious of maintaining your relationship and this takes work and a willingness on your part to do things which you may not initially feel comfortable doing. If the maintenance of a relationship could be reduced to one integral component, then that component would be communication. Whatever issues you are facing with your significant other, communication is the key to understanding. It is best to listen to your partner and be prepared to act on their needs before clearly telling your partner what things you may find difficult and why. At least this opens up a bridge between you and allows for compromises to be made. This is a two way process and you need to also listen to your partners needs and find a way of both parties being content. Relationships are not static entities, they evolve and change as people change (get older, lose jobs, get jobs, have children etc). Relationships, therefore, cannot be assumed to just be fine. One of the ways you may consider compromising is with the home space — if it is shared with your partner. You may find it difficult to always share this space if the other person is watching television programmes you hate or music that you don't enjoy. It is best to discuss this with your partner and try to compromise on the space. For instance you could have a designated time for yourself in a particular room or part of the house where you listen to your music or do whatever activity you enjoy, or you could use headphones as a way of listening or watching things on your laptop while still sharing the space with your partner.

3.6 Peer pressure and cliques

For many of us trying to find our way in the social world is made easier when we find others that we feel are like minded. This may be a very positive and rewarding experience but it may also mean recognising and dealing with peer pressure. This is especially true for people who are in school. Secondary school in particular is a space where hierarchies are formed, there are the 'emo' kids, 'the nerdy kids' etc. Finding your own niche in this space may involve you wanting to be part of a group. You may feel that a particular group is into the same things as you — be it music, fashion or lifestyle. Or some may gravitate towards the 'outcast' group because it is less challenging, emotionally safer, and a chance to be part of a group. This is not necessarily a positive choice however, as it is predicated on a negative view of yourself rather than positively trying to interact with peers.

It is also important to be aware of peer pressure. Do not feel that being encouraged to bully others, shoplift or 'mitch' school are necessary for you to fit in. It is the usual order of things that some people will try to put others down in order to promote themselves in the social hierarchy and it is best to try not to be part of this.

Cliques may exist in any environment from school to college to the work place. Cliques in general are not always a negative thing — that is to say that they may just be a group of like-minded people who enjoy a particular activity. If you find yourself outside of a clique this may be difficult, however. It is best to not assume that you should be part of this type of group or to change yourself in order to try and fit in with it.

3.7 Fashion and identity

Whether you have any interest in fashion or not, the fact remains that it is something which surrounds us in everyday life, from clothes to music to cars. It is intimately linked with our identities and many people choose to express their individuality or their belonging to a particular group through the clothes they wear (an example of this would be Goths who dress in black). It is perfectly understandable to want to express your individuality from any group and it is important to recognise the response you may get from others based on the clothes you wear. So, for example, if you are in college and you attend in a three piece suit you may get attention for this which is likely to be both positive and negative. If you prefer to try and 'fit in' with what others are wearing around you, then just observe what others are wearing and try and find similar clothes when shopping. However, for many people with AS there is a sensory imperative to the clothes they wear, so if certain clothes make you itchy or make you feel uncomfortable in any way then its best to try and source more comfortable clothing. There is a massive variety and choice in terms of clothing now, so it should be relatively straightforward through local shops or the internet if necessary to find suitable (and fashionable — if it is important to you) clothing. It is difficult to shop ethically in terms of clothing but there are a few ethical clothing shops emerging throughout the country. If you cannot afford these clothes you may consider buying in charity shops as they recycle clothes and your money goes towards a good cause. Finding an identity as expressed through your clothing is an evolving process as fashion is driven by corporate imperatives and so is changing ever more quickly. What is fashionable today may be out of fashion in a matter of months — and will also probably be in fashion again in the next few years! (So holding onto those pastel skinny leg trousers may be worth your while!).

3.8 Masturbation and pornography

For most people, the expression of their sexual identity is very important to them. Whether you are straight, gay, lesbian or transgender, you have an equal right to express your sexuality (though unfortunately society may not tolerate all equally). Regardless of your sexuality you are likely to have sexual feelings, though it may be difficult for you to express this sexuality if, for example, you do not have a partner or you live with family. In this situation many people use masturbation as a physical way of expressing sexual feelings or thoughts. This is nothing to be ashamed of or embarrassed by, it is a natural way of expressing these feelings or thoughts. It is important however to try to be conscious of those who share your living space because it is not acceptable to masturbate publicly or in front of others (unless in the context of an agreed act with a partner). It is advisable to lock the door of the room while you are masturbating (for your own privacy and for the sake of others) and to clean up after yourself if required.

Please bear in mind that is best not to bring up masturbation as a topic of conversation at the dinner table. This is not because it is anything to be ashamed of, but rather it is a private matter, if you need reassurance around masturbation or need to talk about it with someone, then choose someone you can trust and ask to speak to them privately. This may be your General Practitioner, a trusted family member, Counsellor or other relevant professional you may be in contact with.

Many people use pornography as a means of stimulation for masturbation. If you are using pornography in this way (on your own or as part of a couple) then it is best to not leave it lying around in your room or especially in shared spaces. Be aware of offending others who may view pornography differently to you (as is their right). While pornography is very widely used it is very important to note that it does not portray real relationships and is not reflective of real life in terms of the types of sexual relationships depicted. Attitudes in pornography are often sexist and disrespectful towards women in particular. Some pornography, such as those featuring children, violent crime or bestiality is illegal to possess and there may be criminal consequences for those caught doing so.

Pornography is also a business. It generates revenue for those who make it and participate in it. It is important to bear in mind that the people taking part are actors being paid to have sex with each other. It is not an educational tool, nor is it representative of the sexual lives of most people. It is performance-based and depicts loveless encounters which are used to titillate and make money. Given the absence of comprehensive sex education in Ireland many adolescents in particular turn to pornography as a way of stimulating, and educating themselves. A further complication for many adolescents with AS is that a lack of peer contact may mean that they have no one to discuss issues around sex with as well as being less likely to learn about sex from knowledgeable, trustworthy sources such as through sex education in school.

3.9 Sex, sexuality and intimacy

If you are in a relationship with someone, then it is likely that sex and intimacy are part of that relationship. If you are in a new relationship or are in a first relationship with someone then the transition into a sexual relationship is an exciting and possibly scary one. In common with relationships generally, it is best to make communication central to the physical side of your relationship. For example, there may be sensory issues for you around touch, the sensation of skin brushing against skin or indeed sex itself. If there are, then speak with your partner about them. It is better to have this conversation than try and avoid intimate sexual situations as this may make your partner feel confused or hurt by your seeming lack of interest.

It is your right to express your sexuality and there may be ways you and your partner can enjoy intimacy through exploration and discussion. This exploration and discussion may happen during sexual activity as a way of finding mutual enjoyment. Try to make it fun and an adventure for both you and your partner. Talking during sex may be arousing and be much easier than talking about sex when not having sex. The choice of words (anatomical, colloquial, crude) is important, for example, crude might be sexy in the moment while childish words may be a big turn-off, or the exact opposite. Listening to your partner's choice of words is important as well as checking in with them to make sure they are comfortable in any given sexual or intimate situation.

Many people with AS like routine as it allows for a certain level of certainty in a generally uncertain world. This is however not always appropriate in the sexual context. The strict adherence to a certain routine may not be what your partner wants, so it is important to have an open communication between both partners and a willingness to try new things. Change is not always a bad thing and when we look at our lives change is inevitable. In the context of a sexual relationship, change can certainly be a good thing as it can often reinvigorate a relationship and provide a new excitement and impetus. Just be prepared to listen and be open to trying new things.

Relationships or sexual encounters with others are not always long term or indeed are not always viewed the same way by both parties. Many sexual encounters are what we may term one night stands — i.e. it is a tryst between sexual partners for only one night. One night stands usually occur between people who do not know each other well (and/or do not want to have a relationship with each other) and may in fact have only met on the day/night as they have a sexual encounter. There are a few rules worth considering should you find yourself in this situation:

- Always use barrier contraception such as a condom as the

pill does not prevent Sexually Transmitted Diseases, do not rely on the other person for this — take responsibility for it yourself

- Barrier contraception is necessary in the prevention of pregnancy and in the spread of sexually transmitted diseases
- One night stands or short term relationships are often felt differently by both parties — one person may want a longer more committed relationship than the other
- It is best to be honest about this from the beginning, so for example if you do not wish to see the person again you could say that you like the person and enjoyed the night but do not wish to be in a relationship
- Do not use sex as a way of getting people to like you or feeling more part of a clique. Only have sex with someone if you are fully consenting

Misunderstandings around the desires of both parties in a short term relationship or a one night stand may have emotional repercussions for one or both. If one party prefers to have just one night with someone, for example, but the other person would prefer a relationship then this can cause confusion and emotional pain. As mentioned previously, it is best to discuss this openly with the other person before you have spent the night together or indeed when it is clear to you that is what the other person wants. It is unlikely (though not impossible) that the first person you have a one night stand or short term relationship with will be 'the one'. Be patient, try and expand your social circle and value yourself.

3.10 Consent

Consent may be defined as a mutual and willing agreement to something between two or more people. In the context of a sexual relationship or a sexual encounter, consent is extremely important. Consent is not a decision that one person decides on in any sexual act, it is mutually agreed. Many people with AS have had difficulty with this issue as they have felt that they have received the right signals from someone (though that 'someone' may not agree) or they may feel sexually frustrated and may physically touch someone without consent. This can have serious consequences legally and emotionally for both parties. It is best to always seek consent and if you do not know the person then it is not appropriate to touch them sexually. It is also equally important that you are consenting to a sexual or physical encounter with someone. As stated above, peer pressure or pressure from a potential sexual partner may make you feel obliged to have a sexual encounter. Ultimately however, do not feel pressurised into it — only engage in a sexual encounter if you are sure you want to and always use contraception. A good reference tool in terms of consent and expectations in sexual relations is www.mwaves.org/. If you have been a victim of sexual assault or rape then it is vital that you speak to someone you can trust and report the incident to the authorities. It is also extremely important to take into consideration the legal age of sexual consent which is set at seventeen years old in Ireland. If you have sexual intercourse with someone younger than this age then you are performing an illegal activity (it is legally defined as child abuse/assault/rape). If, however, there is a sexual relationship between two 15-year-olds who are boyfriend and girlfriend it is deemed to be illegal though not constituting child abuse.

3.11 Alcohol and other drugs

Alcohol and other drugs have been used (and abused) by humans and other species for millennia. Drugs may be used as stimulants, as ways of being more sociable, as a way of relaxing. It is not the purpose or place of this book to judge the use of drugs one way or another but it would be remiss of us not to acknowledge the widespread use of both legal and illegal drugs. The use of drugs is a personal choice but should be done so with the knowledge of the legal, moral and emotional ramifications. In the context of sexual relations alcohol — in particular — may lower inhibitions. It is advisable that you have someone that you can trust and rely on with you if you are getting drunk in pubs, clubs, parties etc as there are many potential dangers to being drunk around others. One of these dangers is that when you lower your inhibitions you may also become more vulnerable. It is advisable that you take some simple precautions if you have been imbibing or using drugs; it is better to take a taxi or public transport home rather than walking — especially late at night. Have a mobile phone with you and ring family or friends if necessary. Do not go to parties alone if you do not know the people inviting you. If you are going out socialising at night try to let someone know where you are going and with whom before you leave. Make sure you have the contact numbers of friends/family and the cab numbers you need, and that someone has the number of your phone which must be on, charged and have credit. College or a workplace may be spaces where there is a lot of pressure on you to socially conform, to use alcohol or drugs, or to be sexually active.

In the next chapter we will look at school, college and work in more detail and explore ways of negotiating your passage through these spaces, and how to use your strengths and skills to your advantage.

4   School, college and work
(Diarmuid Heffernan)

People with an ASD are exactly that — a person with an autism spectrum disorder. There may be a perception in society that this means that everyone on the autism spectrum is the same. This is not the case and while many people with ASDs may find similar difficulties in areas such as social interaction, it is not always the case. Human beings are a complex and diverse species and having an ASD does not mean that you are not as influenced by the social factors which influence the lives of neurotypicals. So, for example, the type of family you are born into, whether they are supportive or non supportive, whether the family is well off or not, the area you were brought up in, whether you had friends or not, if you were bullied etc, all of these factors shape all of us as human beings regardless of being neurotypical or not. However there are some traits that are common (though not necessarily present in all people with an ASD) amongst people with ASDs, these traits may be advantageous in certain contexts and in certain circumstances.

4.1 School

School, as stated in chapter 2 is often the first real point of social interaction outside of the family. It is also a space where peer comparison happens and where societal hierarchies begin to be formed. For the purposes of this section we will concentrate on secondary school. We do this for a number of reasons — for example the difficulties that many people with ASDs experience generally begin in secondary school. This is because children do not tend to notice difference at a younger age and many people we have spoken to who are on the autism spectrum report that primary school was reasonably okay but secondary school was where any perceived differences became problematic (though some people reported noticing the difference from as young as seven years of age). Secondary school is also where pressure is put on adolescents to conform both by peers and indeed by the schools themselves. It is often possible for an adolescent with an

ASD to be punished on the double for 'unusual' behaviour — both by their peers and by the school itself (or indeed people with ASDs are sometimes bullied and then punished for retaliating, yet the bullying is not recognised). Secondary school is where the choosing of subjects occurs and where examinations on the chosen subjects takes place. You may find yourself having to do subjects that you may not be interested in. This is true of most people regardless of ASD or not. The key to getting through these subjects is trying to find something interesting in each and allowing this to make it easier to study. It is also important to have a study routine which incorporates all of your subjects, try not to only study the subjects you are interested in to the detriment of those you may be less interested in. There may be advantages to being a non neurotypical in terms of your ability to dedicate yourself to a task or routine and to spend the time necessary to study it. In other words adhering to a routine can certainly be to your advantage if you harness it properly.

Schools are institutions and they carry with them rules which all students are expected to adhere to. This may be a good or a bad thing for those who are on the autism spectrum. It may make it easier for you to negotiate the school experience if there are clear rules which you can adhere to, or it can be problematic if you do not agree to or understand the rules (though many people with ASD can accept a rule even if it is illogical and they disagree with it, because rules provide certainty and safety). It is best to try and adhere to school rules even if you do not agree with them. This is because school is potentially fraught with many hurdles and difficulties and it is best to try and minimise these and make your passage through school easier. However you may find that others will break the rules blatantly and you may feel like you need to tell teachers or headmaster if this happens. This is a difficult contextually based decision on your part and all we can do in terms of this book is to point out the pitfalls and advantages of telling the school authorities about wrongdoing. If you do tell the school authorities about wrongdoing you may curry favour (intentionally or not) with them. However you may also become unpopular amongst your school peers who may view you as a 'tell tale' for telling the school authorities. This may be because they feel that there should be solidarity amongst students against the school hierarchy/authorities. Be aware that this may be the case and that there may be repercussions for you for the rest of your time in school (and sometimes the 'tell tale' is punished by teachers as well as students because certain behaviours are seen as part of growing up, e.g. 'boys will be boys'). What you may consider to be blatant rule breaking may be part of finding a place in the social hierarchy for others, that is to say that some pupils will behave badly as a way of fitting in.

A fundamental part of the school experience is the feedback you may get from teachers. This may come in the form of criticism. Criticism is difficult for everyone to take but if you don't understand or accept the criticism it is then best to try to talk to the teacher involved after class or in a one to one situation where you can explain that you do not understand or possibly disagree with it. It is best to do this in a polite way and without confrontation. If you are still unhappy, it may be worthwhile discussing the issue with your parents and/or the headmaster. It is worth noting however, that it may be worth taking whatever value/learning you can from criticism even when it is emotionally or physically painful (or makes you sick), it is generally intended for your benefit not your harm.

Remember school is not an infinite time and space that you are wed to, it is a finite period which only serves as a stepping stone to the rest of your life. Though it may be difficult at times, it is a space you are ultimately passing through rather than stuck in. It may be worth getting involved in hobbies or outside interests, clubs, social groups, music, riding, sports etc as a means of balancing out the school experience and of meeting peers socially outside of the school environment.

4.2 College

Whether you have decided that you want to continue to third level education while in second level education (or in primary school if you are particularly organised!) or if you decide to return to/resume/continue/or begin it is worthwhile to remember that third level is very different from primary or secondary education. It is different in terms of its organisation, its expectations and in terms of the rules and regulations (or indeed lack of routine that you may have been used to in school) attached to colleges. This is important because many people both on the autism spectrum and on the neurotypical spectrum find the transition to college to be challenging and difficult to negotiate. For people on the autism spectrum the rules and regulations of school may be reassuring, having spent years getting used to both the routines of school and indeed the people who inhabit it, it may be very difficult to transition to a new environment with different expectations and a new cohort of people to get used to. One of the reassuring aspects of school may be the presence of the same teachers and classmates over your school years (this may be a case of 'better the devil you know' even if you dislike your teachers or classmates at least you know what to expect — the unknown may appear to be much worse!). These teachers may become trusted advocates on your behalf, in college however, there are new lecturers for different modules in classes that may number into the hundreds. Therefore you may not get any personal attention or have any real interaction with your lecturers. This may or may not be a good thing for you. It may be good in the sense of disappearing into the fabric of college life without having the pressures of being in a smaller classroom and being expected to interact with others. Or it may suit you in the sense that you are only studying subjects that you are interested in rather than ones you are forced to do in the second level curriculum. It may be difficult however if you are not certain what the lecturer wants in terms of assignments, if you need clarification with anything, or if you miss a lecture. College, therefore, is also a potentially challenging space for those on the autism spectrum. It carries both stresses and rewards but may often be necessary as a right of passage or as a means to getting a job.

There are a number of ways of getting into college in Ireland now. One is by completing the Leaving Certificate examination. There are generally between seven and ten subject's studied for the Leaving Certificate (a minimum of six is required) and each subject has a corresponding points total attached to it — which is based on the results given, for example, the most points awarded for a subject would be an 'A' mark decreasing to the least for a 'D'. The Leaving Certificate is further divided into Pass and Honours subject's so each student has a choice between doing a Pass or Honours in each subject. Honours subjects are more comprehensive than Pass subjects and therefore carry more points. Entry to courses in third level education is based on this points system and each third level course has a corresponding point's requirement based on the Leaving Certificate examinations. The Leaving Certificate cycle starts in fifth year in secondary school and continues to sixth year, the Leaving Certificate exams are then held at the end of sixth year. In order to get into the third level course you desire, it may be wise to look at the subjects most pertinent to that course and concentrate on getting good results in them for your Leaving Certificate. For example if you wish to do Mechanical Engineering in Third Level education then maths is a primary element of that course and it will be necessary for you to do well in maths for your Leaving Cert (incidentally higher level maths carries the highest points in the Leaving Cert). Application to college is through the CAO system which can be accessed online (you can view point's tables on this site). Another option may be the DARE scheme. The Disability Access Route to Education (DARE) is a college and university admissions scheme which offers places on a reduced points basis to school leavers under 23 years old with disabilities who have completed an Irish Leaving Certificate (you can look up the DARE scheme online or school guidance counsellors should be able to advise you around this scheme).

You may also apply for third level education as a mature student. This requires that you be 23 years of age or over when applying. In this instance you may be entitled to state grants if you meet the criteria for Back to Education Allowance (this may be accessed if you have been unemployed for 12 months or over and meet the college criteria for entry to a particular course). If you have not completed any formal state exams and are under the age of twenty three you may need to do an access course which will give you the required academic experience. This may take the form of doing a Leaving Certificate in a Post Leaving Certificate College, or doing an evening course in a third level institute.

If you have not completed a Leaving Certificate or have not achieved sufficient Leaving Cert points for a third level course, do not despair. It is very difficult to decide what you want to do with the rest of your life when you are a teenager. It may also be very difficult to contemplate this type of decision if you are finding school stressful because of bullying, intimidation or finding the social aspect difficult. There are options to consider rather than going straight into third level education from secondary school. For example, if you have not finished school and do not want to attend third level institutes, it may be worth considering applying to the National Learning Network (NLN). The National Learning Network is the training and employment division of the Rehab Group and provides accredited training and specialist support to people who are distant from the labour market. Each year, 5,000 people learn and study in the NLN's including many who may otherwise find it difficult to gain employment and to develop the skills to move forward with their careers.

National Learning Network currently offers over 40 different vocational programmes which carry certification and are designed to lead directly to jobs or progression to further education (www.nln.ie/). Please note that the NLN is not a panacea, it does not suit everyone and the courses are generally one to two years, following which you will still have to find employment or get into another course.

If the National Learning Network is not suitable to your needs and/or you do not want to physically attend a college, or you have not found a course that suits you, then it may also be worth considering the Open University. The Open University courses generally require attendance at a set number of tutorials per year but for the vast majority of the course, you are expected to study at home and complete/submit assignments. The Open University also provides courses which may serve as an access to formal third level education.

If you decide to attend third level education then it is worth spending some time picking a discipline that suits you and that you will be interested in. There are a number of criteria to consider when deciding on a course that suits. For example, is it a subject that you are enthused by? Is it a course that will be more likely to get you employment? When choosing, be aware of the years of study involved in completing a third level course. If you are doing a course that you feel will give you a better chance of gaining employment (as opposed to doing a course in which the material enthuses you), then bear in mind this does not necessarily mean that you will enjoy it and may mean working harder than if you were doing a course you are interested in — regardless of the employment opportunities it may give you. In the work section we will look in more detail at the types of jobs that you may be interested in and that may be more suitable for you, and the commensurate courses required to get these jobs.

4.2.1 College issues

Having looked at the possibilities of college and the various permutations regarding courses, other options etc we will now look at the issues you may face if you are about to, or indeed have already started college. If you have a diagnosis of an ASD one of the first things to consider when you are entering or indeed are already in college, is whether to disclose your diagnosis to your fellow students, lecturers, course co-ordinators etc. This is a very personal decision, but there are some issues to contemplate before making a decision around disclosure. For instance not disclosing can lead to many problems which you may be unable to explain to others in isolation, while disclosing may be very helpful to your lecturers in particular in supporting you. An example of this would be group work and we will discuss this in detail later in the text. A further consideration in deciding to disclose or not is the support you will receive from the disability officers in your college if you do disclose. This may be difficult for you to do given the stigma many people feel still exists around the word disability. However, this is a generalised term used to describe difference and should not prevent you from seeking services and supports that may be very useful to you. Finally in contemplating disclosure it is worth considering the positive accumulative effect of disclosure. Put simply, the more people with ASDs that disclose, the more knowledge and understanding amongst staff and fellow students in colleges and the more likelihood of better outcomes for future students with AS. We believe that you can negotiate your way through college if you decide not to disclose (as many students and indeed staff do in third level institutions), but it is possible that it may make that journey more difficult for you.

4.2.2 Group work

Earlier in the text we looked at some of the expectations of college. One of the fundamental aspects of college is the inherent social interactions that take place in the college environment. This does not necessarily mean being forced to talk to other student's, lecturers etc but it does mean that you will be in classes of varying size and this means an inevitable degree of social interaction. Many people with AS prefer to be in bigger classes where they are anonymous and there is no expectation for social interaction with other students in their class. Other people with AS see college as an opportunity to meet people and possibly make friends. Most courses in third level institutions now include group work as an integral part of the college curriculum. Colleges will say that this is to ready people for the work environment where it will usually be necessary to interact with colleagues in a group. Many students might disagree and say it is an easier way to lecture and that they might not necessarily want to be employed in an organisation where group work is expected, but would rather work autonomously/independently. Either way, the fact is that colleges do use group work and it can be a very difficult and demanding aspect of college life, whether you have an ASD or not. If you find yourself having to be part of group as a requirement for your course then it is worth considering talking to your lecturer or the course co-ordinator and discussing the challenges that group work may pose for you. This may involve disclosure as discussed previously. If you have not disclosed then it may be important to be part of a group where you are friends with, or familiar with the group members or a group member. If this is not possible, then it is important to try and negotiate with the group in terms of the direction/purpose of the group project and then to decide who does what in terms of the different pieces of work that are required. This is often a difficult negotiation requiring a degree of compromise. Even if you feel that your way of looking at a topic is the right way and the group have decided to do it a different way, bear in mind that group work gives you the opportunity to practice your negotiation skills as well as learning to compromise. This is not to say that the work itself is not important but rather the dynamic of the group is at least equally important. It is worth noting that many groups have members who designate themselves as leader, and members who do less than others. This is often part of the difficulty with group work and it is best not to get too concerned with the division of labour (unless you are being overworked or excluded).

4.2.3 Public speaking and presentations

College courses often have a presentation requirement to them. This may include presenting individual work or group work. Many people with ASDs enjoy the experience of public speaking because it is scripted, it does not contain the unexpected as most social interaction does, and it allows the individual to showcase their knowledge and ability — which may be difficult to get across in other ways. Public speaking can, however, be nerve-racking for many. Standing in front of groups of people who are all focused on your words can be intimidating. To allay this feeling, it is often helpful to acknowledge your nerves, you might simply say "I find public speaking difficult and I am very nervous, so please bear with me". This is often a way of getting an audience on your side, very few people are totally comfortable with public speaking, therefore the audience will generally empathise with your feelings of nervousness. Other commonly recommended methods of allaying your nerves such as imagining your audience naked may cause you more discomfort or even trauma! But if you have a tried and trusted method that works for you, then do use it.

4.2.4 Managing your own learning

A core component of a successful college experience is being organised. This means getting assignments completed and submitted on time, studying for exams, and deciding on a thesis topic in sufficient time (if a thesis is required for your course). The first step to being organised is to purchase a diary. Begin by writing your timetable into your diary, then include and highlight dates of assignments. If you are not sure of assignment dates, you should approach your lecturer either before or after your classes and ask them. Also include in the diary any other appointments you may have during your college week along with any extra-curricular activities you may be involved with. Include study time in your week and this may also include the time needed to research and write up an assignment. For example, if you finish college at three on Wednesdays, then you could pencil in three hours of study/research/writing time from three to six. The diary supports you in developing a routine and good study habits are best developed in your first year in college rather than trying to play catch up at the end of your college year or in your final college year. The diary may be in physical form or in online form (for example Google calendar is a very useful online tool). It may also be worth putting in your diary the contact numbers of your lecturer/tutor/PA to the department etc to check dates or explain absence or late submission.

If you decide to disclose and receive the support of the disability office in your college then they may be able to support you in the organisational aspect of college. There are also learning support offices in most colleges which have a remit to support students with specific and general learning requirements. This would include organisational skills, study skills and submitting assignments. Most colleges now require students to submit both a paper copy of assignments and an e-copy. Though there is some general tuition available to support students to use online submission through college IT departments, this is often difficult to follow, in stuffy crowded rooms and may not always suit students in terms of clashing with classes. Therefore it is often worthwhile getting the assistance of the learning support office. If you have not, or do not want to access the support of the learning support office, most colleges have an orientation day for individual classes and these may be very helpful in familiarising yourself with your campus and also where to go if you do have IT difficulties for example.

A further key element of college life is completing assignments and studying for exams. We include these two elements together in this section as they both involve similar methods of study/research. The first step to consider when looking at an assignment is asking what is this assignment looking for? What is it asking? And how do I answer it? The next step is to begin to research relevant books, and focus on individual chapters that may be relevant. If you can afford the cost of photocopying then it may be worth photocopying these chapters, reading them, then highlighting important passages or words. If you cannot afford to photocopy then learning support officers often have access to photocopying facilities, alternatively save the important pieces onto a memory stick or write into a notebook and remember to keep the reference to the book you got the notes from including the author and the title as it will make it much easier to look up and take in afterwards. When you have sufficient research done then you may consider beginning to write your assignment, (you can consider using Endnote, Zotero etc, any manual system may be useful).

The same principles apply to studying for exams. It may be worthwhile looking at past exam papers (these may be available on request or accessed through online media such as Blackboard etc) for clues as to what may come up in your exams, and it may also be a good way of practising exam papers. If you are beginning to study a subject for exams it is worth going through your reading list, picking out books and chapters that are relevant and then photocopying, highlighting etc as per assignments advice previously in this text. It is again very important to consider the time aspect of this type of study. It is generally very time consuming so it is extremely important to use your diary as a way of creating the time you need in order to do this work. We advise against trying to do this work two nights before your exams start! Allow plenty of time, begin to use the diary when you start college, and use it to develop good study habits and routines from the outset. A number of people with AS find it difficult to maintain concentration on a given subject when trying to study. One way of trying to address this difficulty is by having music on in the background as it can serve to stimulate or alternatively block out distracting sensory stimuli. Another method of maintaining concentration is to divide study time into manageable blocks of, for example, a half hour or hour — then take a break and do something you enjoy for the same period of time (some people recommend taking a walk outside to get some air, others use the time for 'gaming') before returning to study for another half hour/hour. In this way it may be possible to get a reasonable amount of study done while keeping your concentration levels high. It is also worth trying to extend the amount of time spent studying while gradually decreasing the amount of time spent on leisure.

If you find the idea of doing an exam in a very crowded room with hundreds of other students is creating anxiety for you and if you have disclosed to the disability department of your college you can request to do your exams in a separate exam room with a small number of others (or sometimes on your own). This may serve to alleviate some of the stress you may feel about doing the exam.

You may also request an extra amount of time to do your exam if in a separate room.

4.2.5 Sensory issues

We have dealt with the sensory issues many people with ASDs may feel in certain spaces throughout this book but it is pertinent to state here that college spaces also contain many of the sensory issues of other spaces — and sometimes even more. Small classrooms filled with students may contain sights, sounds and smells that are problematic for you. This is difficult to get around due to the pragmatics involved in college education. We would recommend (if it is possible) that you familiarise yourself with the campus you will be attending and the building your classes are going to be held in before you start as a way of having a sense of what lies ahead of you (for example, projectors, L.E.lights, air-conditioning, nearby noisy classes etc).

This also applies to your mode of transport to and from college. It is best to contemplate how you will get to and from your chosen campus. For example bus, train etc. If you find it uncomfortable to take the bus due to sensory or other issues then it may be worth considering cycling or walking to and from campus. Either way it is good practice to familiarise yourself with the route to campus and the method of transport that best suits you. You could do so by practising journeys, find classrooms, buildings, go to campus in advance and without time pressure, so that you are familiar with location and timing before doing it under pressure. If you do have to take a train or bus them look at timetables and there may be a way of travelling to and from campus at less busy times. You may also find that using headphones with relaxing music/music that makes you happy or reassuring words/music can alleviate some of the sensory difficulties you may experience on a bus or train (others may bring books or magazines or possibly listen to or watch media on I-Pads etc — please use headphones if doing so!).

4.2.6 Accommodation in college

Part of the college experience for many involves moving out of home for the first time and sharing accommodation with others.

We have previously looked at the do's and don'ts of sharing a space with others, but it is worth taking into consideration issues like living on your own, if you would prefer to share a space with others or if you would prefer to live alone. Either choice carries monetary implications as living alone will generally be more expensive than sharing, however sharing may bring issues of conflict/difficulty in terms of compromising fitting in with others — and they with you. If you do decide to share it is worth considering how many people you may share with. Further general considerations include how close to campus you want to live, the possibility of house parties in the house/apartment you share! If the possibility of a house party occurring in your shared accommodation fills you with anxiety it may be possible to find a house share with older students (Masters/PHD) who may be less inclined towards house parties etc. Alternatively have an agreement with your co-habitors around when a hose party may occur, making certain parts of the house/flat off limits to others at the party (if you attend the party you may want to escape to your room for some time to ground yourself or take a break from the noise) and agreeing on cleaning up responsibilities. Learning how to cook and shop for yourself are both integral aspects of life which we will deal with in chapter six of this book.

4.2.7 Research

Much modern research can begin online, either through your own searches or through college search engines/library search engines. This means that you often begin research on your personal computer or college computer. However, you will usually need to use the library as a resource to find in-depth academic research. Most colleges will include a library tour in their student orientation day and this may be a very useful way of familiarising yourself with the physical space and the mechanics of using the library. Alternatively the disability office on campus may be able to provide you with a tour or give you useful tips on the layout and use of the library. If you find yourself having difficulty in using the library, and don't want to use the disability office, then it may be worthwhile approaching library staff and asking for their assistance. Library staff are usually very pleased to assist library users.

4.2.8 College administration requirements

Like every institution there are a certain amount of bureaucratic requirements attached to college life. We do not mean this in a negative way, rather in a realistic way. The submission of assignments requires an e-copy, for example, but there are other aspects to college administration that you will need to interact with. The grants system would be one example of this. The Government have promised a reform of the grants system to streamline it and make it more fit for purpose. However, most students find that their grants appear to arrive ad hoc without any way of finding out when they are due to arrive. The best advice we can give here is try to be patient! Arguing or getting annoyed with college staff who are not responsible for any delay will not make it any easier or make the grant arrive more quickly. It is best to check in with the grants office by phone regarding the grants.

4.2.9 The social potential of college

To finish this section we will look at the potential for college to provide a social network or social opportunities for you as a student. Most colleges have a variety of societies which focus on niche group interests. These may run the gamut from mainstream sports such as hurling, soccer and rugby to more 'minority' sports such as Frisbee. There are generally also role playing societies, gaming societies, mountaineering societies etc. These societies provide a potential opportunity for you to join a club focused around a niche interest of yours and can be a really useful way of getting to know like-minded people, make friends and to view college from a different perspective. Despite the fact that college is centred on learning, it is also a place where social interaction can be practised and friendships can be made. It may also be a place where many form long term relationships/friendships or life partners. It can become problematic for many people with ASDs if they only focus on going to college to study a course/subject as college as a space is intrinsically a social space and contain the challenges of all social spaces in it. Therefore it is very difficult to complete a college course without interacting with others, and we suggest that it is best to try and view this positively as an opportunity, rather than see it as an added burden to being in college.

4.3 Work

4.3.1 Introduction

Having an ASD can be an advantage in life. Many people with AS are more focused on a task or topic, and may be less susceptible to group-think or to put it another way, they have the ability to 'think outside the box'. The objectivity of standing outside potential group thinking allows for a different perspective which other consensus seekers may overlook (Dr Temple Grandin and her work around building cattle corrals is a prime example of this quality, where she is able to see what the animals see and design for them). People with ASD may be more honest both in their endeavours and their interactions, or may pay more attention to details that neurotypicals may find boring or monotonous. In general people with ASD are capable of doing the same work as anyone else is, you may however be drawn to certain types of work that coincide with your own passions or interests, or work that may allow you to work alone without having to be part of a group.

There may also be disadvantages to having an ASD (one of which is the stereotyping of people with ASDs as being geniuses). If your workplace is bright and noisy, then it may prove to be a sensory hell to work in, with so many distractions that it is impossible to focus on your work. Offices can be difficult spaces to fit in with colleagues for everyone but especially if you find social interaction difficult. Being overly fixed on a routine or task can be disadvantageous if you are asked to be flexible and move on to another task or to move outside of your comfort zone geographically or in terms of the work. This may be especially true if you are very proficient and reliable in your work, as you may be promoted. Management or promotion usually involve the management or supervision of others and this would mean more social interaction and more expectation that you understand others perspective.

The key here is to find out what you are good at and try to maximise this. Finding something you are passionate about and trying to make a career out of it is a sensible thing to do. If however you cannot find a career that matches your interests then it is best to look at your qualities, what you find difficult and what you are good at. Therefore if you are good at sequential organising but find social interaction as part of a team very difficult then, for example, a job in a library may be worth pursuing (some people might feel that this is stereotyping but there in our experience many people with ASDs do enjoy working in a library).

Work may also provide the opportunity to develop a social network or friendships. It is also not uncommon for people to meet a romantic partner through work (this is not a given obviously but it is certainly a possibility). Work is also a way of having a focus, of providing you with intellectual and social stimulation. It provides money, which may not be an end in itself for you, but may provide you with a means by which to live independently, free from the financial supports from others. The first step when contemplating work is to think of a job that may suit you. It may be then worthwhile looking at where that job might be and before you apply to a company it may be worth thinking about the practicalities of working there, such as, transport to and from the place of employment. This may be problematic if the only way to get to and from work is by bus for example but you may have sensory or other issues around being on a bus (we have some suggestions on how to deal with sensory difficulties on buses or trains in the college section). This does not mean you should not apply for the job but rather take into consideration the practicalities if you get the job and what these might mean for you. If the bus is too difficult to take then look at the possibilities of cycling or walking there, or could you rent an apartment or house nearby. If you are comfortable with the practical steps of potentially getting to and from a specific geographical location (be it city, town etc) for a job then the next step is to look at how you may get that job.

4.3.2 Curriculum Vitae

Before applying for a job you should have an up-to-date Curriculum Vitae (CV). This is a document which charts your previous relevant work experience, as well as your college or school results, and your interests and achievements. There are many templates for drawing up a CV online or if you prefer to interact with someone it may be worth dropping in to your local FAS office and seeking their advice on how to best present your

CV (third level colleges generally have a careers guidance office which may be able to give you advice or support also). It is best to tailor your CV for whatever job you may be applying for by accentuating the previous relevant experience, and interests that you may have which are relevant to the job you are applying for.

4.3.3 Job interviews

Job interviews may be nerve-racking experiences for many especially those with an ASD. Many job interviews now have a panel rather than just a single interviewer which may be more intimidating for you. There are some simple steps to approaching a job interview which may be very helpful in making it a less nerve-racking experience. It is best to be early for the interview (not two hours early!), fifteen minutes before you are due to be interviewed should be sufficient time to acclimatise with your environment. Plan your route before you do the interview (you could use Google Maps, Google Earth etc). Look at what mode of transport you will need to take in order to get there before the interview, consult timetables etc in case of different times on different days, and practice it before the day of the interview so you know exactly how long it will take. Also take into consideration which mode of transport you are most comfortable with. If you feel more comfortable walking or cycling, bear in mind that it does not generally leave a good impression with prospective employers if you are sweating profusely after your exertions! In general it is best to have a neat appearance for your interview, wear a tie, shoes and slacks if they do not cause you sensory discomfort (or find smart clothes that don't cause sensory discomfort). It is also best to shower and shave before the interview. It may well be worthwhile learning relevant information about the company before you do the interview, so that you are fore-armed against any such questions. Be concise in answering the questions you are asked but try not to give yes and no answers, elaborate where necessary but do not over-elaborate. If you do not understand a question you are asked, then you can ask politely for the interviewee to rephrase the question.

If you have gotten as far as interview, then you are a valid candidate and are as worthy a candidate as anyone else. Many people with an ASD struggle with whether to disclose their diagnosis to an employer or not. It is very difficult to objectively assess whether disclosure will work to your advantage or not as it is very much dependent on individual perspective employers. If you have decided to tell your potential employer then a job interview is a place that you may decide to do so. If you do decide to tell, then it may be best to say it at the end of the interview and to accentuate the positive aspects of being a person with an ASD, for instance as your diligence, honesty and good work ethic.

4.3.4 Working with others

If you have handed in your CV, done your job interview and have been employed by a company, what are the issues you may face? As with school, college and many other areas of life, a primary aspect of working life is the interaction with others that is required. This is an area that many people with an ASD may find extremely difficult, and in fact may be the most challenging aspect of working life. There are some guidelines to consider as regards interacting with work colleagues. The first is to try and engage with your work colleagues. This can mean something as simple as asking someone how their weekend was, or whether they planned anything nice for their coming weekend. You may view this as small talk but as discussed previously in this book, it is sometimes an expectation that you would interact in this way with others (even if you do not seem to be saying anything that you consider meaningful or important). Part of the expectation in many workplaces is to be part of a team. This is something to consider before you decide to take this type of job. If you do decide to take a job that involves working as part of a team (similarly to group work in college) it will involve a negotiation and possibly some compromise in order to make it work. It is also best to try and find value in everyone's contribution, even if you do not agree with it. You can express this verbally through phrases like: 'I understand your perspective but I saw it this way...' This promotes a constructive conversation where the other person still feels their contribution is valued and it also allows you to give your perspective. If you are too blunt or are perceived as too critical you may find your interactions with colleagues become more difficult as they may not respond positively to the bluntness or criticism.

Depending on where you work, there may be an expectation that you socialise with your work colleagues. You might view this as either an opportunity to make friends/get to know your colleagues better, or you may find the idea of this type of social interaction to be anxiety-inducing. This may be especially true if you are exhausted by a long day of work and/or interacting with others, and your 'social batteries' may be low from the effort. If you decide to socialise with your colleagues all the social expectations of any interaction apply: do not disclose very personal information about yourself, allow others to talk about their interests, and do not spend too much time discussing your own interests. Be prepared to broaden the palette of conversational topics. Sometimes a way of doing this is by listening and observing what others are discussing. Often times a way of reducing your social discomfort might be to ask the other person questions as a way of showing interest in the others point of view. You can do so by asking general questions and stimulating conversation, most people react positively to being given the opportunity to talk about themselves or their lives/interests.

Be aware that many offices contain 'office banter'. This may include potentially insulting comments made in a joking manner between colleagues. Be aware that this is often a unique culture to each place of employment that may have built up over a number of years. You may not like what is being said, or you may feel you need to join in to be accepted by others but it is best to observe this and listen to what is being said. Do not feel pressurised into partaking in office banter if you do not feel comfortable about it. For instance, a nickname used between two colleagues who know each other well may be inappropriate when used by someone new, as can over-familiar or sexually suggestive terms. Sexist words (eg 'pet', 'doll' or 'girl') are best avoided even when everyone else appears to be using them. If you do decide to join in be aware of the unique and individual tolerances of each person for different types of humour, and also consider the fact that many of your colleagues may know each other for a long time and have built up a rapport and trust that allows for comments etc that may cause offence if said by others. For example it is best not to launch into sexual innuendo (even of others are doing so) if you are new in a workplace.

4.3.5 Responding to managers

You may feel that you know more about your work than your manager does, and as well as this they may ask you to carry out tasks that you may not agree with. This is the prerogative of management and it is best to carry out your tasks if asked to do so (unless the task is demeaning, dangerous or could be construed as bullying). Despite the fact that you may not agree with them, they are still the manager and — especially if you enjoy the job — it is best to do as you are asked. If you are unsure as to what your manager requires of you, then it is reasonable to politely ask them to repeat the instruction and to clarify it. If you have told the manager about your ASD then you may be able to ask them to explain in writing or by e mail as well as presenting it to you verbally. A written task is often more easily understood, or, you can read it in your own time without feeling under the pressure you may feel if it is presented to you verbally.

4.3.6 Job duties and promotion

Most jobs come with a list of duties, which are essentially the tasks that your position requires. In most cases these duties will require a degree of flexibility from the employee. This means that you may be asked to do other duties outside of the named ones on your job description from time to time — or as your job evolves (many new job contracts include a caveat that the employee may need to carry out other tasks outside of their named duties as required by management). It is best to be aware of this when you apply for a job, and it is worthwhile reading through your contract thoroughly. It is best to try to carry out whatever duties your employer requests of you (again, within reason as stipulated above).

Many people with an ASD, given the opportunity, make honest and diligent employees. This may mean promotion. Promotion is a recognition of your abilities as a worker, to do the tasks required of you efficiently and proficiently. It is not necessarily a recognition of your ability to lead, manage or motivate others, yet these are very often the requirements of a supervisory or management position if you are promoted. Managing others is often a difficult task, it involves empathy, hard work, discipline and patience, amongst many other traits. If you do get offered a promotion to a management position, bear these requirements in mind. It will often involve a change in your tasks or an increase in tasks and will almost certainly include more responsibility.

4.3.7 Recognising harassment

This may be a tricky area for someone with an ASD. We previously discussed 'office banter' and how this may be a culture in many places of work (not just offices). However there are limits to what is acceptable for each of us as individuals regarding what we consider to be a joke, or what we consider to be offensive. If you are unsure what constitutes banter and what constitutes harassment it is advisable to talk to a trusted confidant about it and use examples. This will serve to share the difficulty you are experiencing with someone — i.e. 'a problem shared is a problem halved' — as well as getting an objective opinion.

4.3.8 Harassment and employment rights

Citizens Information describes harassment in the following way:

The Employment Equality Acts 1998-2011 place an obligation on all employers to prevent harassment in the workplace. Under this law, you are entitled to bring a claim to the Equality Tribunal and your employer may be obliged to pay you compensation if you are harassed by reason of your:

- Gender
- Civil status
- Family status, for example, as a parent of a child
- Sexual orientation
- Age
- Disability
- Race
- Religious belief
- Membership of the Traveller community

Harassment based on any of the above grounds is a form of discrimination in relation to conditions of employment. The Employment Equality Acts 1998-2011 define harassment as "unwanted conduct" which is related to any of the 9 discriminatory grounds above. Sexual harassment is any form of "unwanted verbal, non-verbal or physical conduct of a sexual nature". In both cases it is defined as conduct which "has the purpose or effect of violating a person's dignity and creating an intimidating, hostile, degrading, humiliating or offensive environment for the person" and it is prohibited under the Acts.

The "unwanted conduct" includes spoken words, gestures or the production and display of written words, pictures and other material. This includes offensive gestures or facial expressions, unwelcome and offensive calendars, screen-savers, e-mails and any other offensive material.

Bullying at work when it is related to one of the discriminatory grounds is covered by the Employment Equality Acts. Harassment and bullying at work which is not linked to a discriminatory ground is a health and safety issue.

Harassment can be by a fellow worker, your boss or someone in a superior position, a client, a customer or any other employment contact. Harassment can take place at work or on a training course, on a work trip, at a work social event or any other occasion connected with your job.

Under the Acts, your employer may also be held responsible if harassment takes place outside the course of your employment but you are treated differently at work because of your rejection or acceptance of the harassment. If you bring a claim under the Acts, you cannot then be subjected to victimisation at work in retaliation for making your claim.

Your employer should have a policy and procedures to deal with and prevent harassment at work. The policy should set out what is unacceptable behaviour at work. An effective grievance or complaints procedure should be in place to deal with complaints about harassment. All employees must be aware of the policy and procedures. The "Code of Practice on Sexual Harassment and Harassment at Work" aims to give practical guidance to employers and employees.

4.3.9 Employment rights of people with disabilities

Employees with disabilities have the same employment rights as other employees.

Equality legislation: The Employment Equality Acts 1998-2011 outlaw discrimination on the grounds of disability in employment, including training and recruitment. However the Employment Equality Acts state that an employer is not obliged to recruit or retain a person who is not fully competent or capable of undertaking the duties attached to a job. If you have a mental health difficulty the Equality Authority has published a booklet, Equality and mental health: how the law can help you (www.equality.ie/).

Reasonable accommodation: The Employment Equality Acts 1998-2011 require employers to take reasonable steps to accommodate the needs of employees and prospective employees with disabilities. Reasonable accommodation can be defined as some modification to the tasks or structure of a job or workplace, which would allow the qualified employee with a disability to fully do the job and enjoy equal employment opportunities. However, under EU legislation, employers are not obliged to provide special treatment or facilities if the cost of doing so is excessive or disproportionate.

The above information is available on the Citizens Information website (www.citizensinformation.ie/) which is an excellent source of information on all of your rights and entitlements as an employee.

4.3.10 Employee Assistance Programmes

There are many schemes to assist people back into employment such as the Employer Based Training (EBT) scheme, the JobBridge scheme or the Work Placement Programme, all of which involve internships with willing employers for those receiving welfare payments from the state including Disability payments. For further information on any of these schemes refer to the citizens advice website or contact the Department of Social Protection.

A further potential option for employment for people with ASDs is Specialisterne. Specialisterne, which translates from Danish as "the specialists", is a social enterprise providing assessment, training, education and IT consultancy services, where most of the employees are people with autism. It is currently setting up a franchise in Ireland based in the Dublin offices of software company SAP and is already working with Microsoft and Accenture on employment opportunities. See ie.specialisterne.com/ for more information.

If you are already in employment there are organisations such as EmployAbility which assist people with a disability who are job ready and need a level of support to succeed in long-term and sustainable employment. In the next chapter we will begin by looking at sensory issues before discussing the many other day to day issues you may experience.

5 Planning *(Stuart Neilson)*

Some people appear to have a rare ability to hold all their tasks, appointments and shopping lists in their heads. Most of us do not. Some of us can barely leave the house without going through something like an airline preflight-check (Is the gas off? The back door locked? Am I fully clothed? Where am I going?). Whichever end of this continuum you match, planning tasks and keeping clear notes is **always** going to help, even when you think you can hold it all in your head. We have excellent long-term memories compared to any other species, but limited short-term memory — every extra item that you are thinking about can add to anxiety and difficulty remembering every other item, and this is especially so when responding to a change in plan.

5.1 Obstacles to getting things done

There are four main sets of obstacles to getting things done — obstacles to getting started, obstacles to staying on task, obstacles to completing tasks and (perhaps most importantly) difficulty in regulating activity.

Obstacles to getting started include inertia, lack of motivation, being overwhelmed by complexity and feeling that there is no time left after other more urgent demands. Obstacles to staying on task include sensory distractions, lack of focus, a disorganised workplace, difficulty switching tasks when disturbed and difficulty coping with unexpected problems or changes. Obstacles to completion include unrealistic expectations, fear of mistakes or criticism, perfectionism and unrealistic comparison with others. A lack of regulation, or poor moderation, of stimulation and activity leads to cycles of over-stimulation and enthusiastic over-working followed by burnout and unproductive tiredness.

There are some very specific neurological factors related to autism spectrum disorder that feature in all of these obstacles.

Executive function is the set of cognitive processes that oversee planning of motor movements and sequences of actions, short-term working memory, maintain appropriate attention, solve problems, verbal reasoning, moderate impulses and manage to switching between tasks. Poor executive function (or executive dysfunction) can accompany high verbal skills or high IQ, and can be extremely difficult to pinpoint in an otherwise academic or accomplished individual.

Sensory processing disorders include hyper- and hyposensitivity as well as sensory integration dysfunction and synaesthesia. Sensory hypersensitivity means being overly sensitive, typically to sound or light. Hypersensitivity can make a busy workplace or library a very uncomfortable environment to study or get things done in. Sensory hyposensitivity means being under-responsive, typically to exercise, gravity (vestibular sense), being unaware of your own body's location (proprioception) or to tactile sensations. Hyposensitivity can make you slower to get started at the beginning of the day, liable to tripping or bumping into objects and less aware of injuries. Disorders of sensory integration mean that the various senses are not integrated with each other, or with the control of motor and other functions. Synaesthesia is the perception of one sense when a different sense is stimulated — for instance seeing coloured numbers or letters, or sensing aroma from images. Synaesthesia can be a very rich and rewarding experience, but it may also contribute to dyslexia and dyscalculia or slow down the processing of material.

A third neurological effect is perseveration or obsessiveness. A major difference between perseveration in autism and perseveration in, for instance, obsessive-compulsive disorder, is that the obsessive interests are the source of pleasure rather than distress, often very intense pleasure. Sometimes you may find that *"you don't see the wood for the trees"* — you are extremely good with details, especially that details that fascinate you, but not so good at perceiving the overall plans and objectives. You may also derail the flow of a discussion into tangents related to minutiae that nobody else seems to care about. It is also entirely natural to you to assume that everyone else pursued the same tangent as you, at the same time, because that is the way you perceived the flow of the discussion — so it can be quite a surprise or shock to discover that they are still firmly on the old topic and possibly quite annoyed with your detour. Obsession can be positive — an eye for detail and an intense drive can be very powerful motivations to succeed when your own interests and your tasks are aligned.

A final neurological effect is one that is often termed a *lack of social imagination*, a difficulty in coping with situations in which the outcome is either unknown or too complicated to predict. Many people are happy to dive into the unknown and actually enjoy the thrill of the unexpected, or meeting strangers for the first time. You may find a situation with an unknown outcome very hard, especially when it involves people you are less familiar with. This might be something as simple as how long a visitor will stay or something as complicated as what a holiday abroad will be like.

Success is its own motivator — if you like jam, then there is nothing so satisfying as seeing a shelf-full of your own home-made jam. Many of the things that we do are not so visual, but there are methods to turn achievement into lists and other visual records of successful achievement.

5.1.1 Getting things started

Getting things started is hard for most people, but some of us find it harder than others. Realising that other people — often visibly successful achievers — have difficulty getting started can help you start too, especially if they share their tips for getting on with things. One of the biggest tips of all is that a lot of achievement is not much fun, and some achievement is heartbreakingly painful, or even heartbreakingly boring. If you were to collect an accurate record of how you have spent all your time last year, much of it was probably spent on things that do not matter any more, and never will matter. A great deal of time was probably spent on revision topics that never came up in tests, the answers you rehearsed for questions that were never asked or the records that you prepared for a boss who then had more important things to deal with — and these things that took time away from the revision topics that were examined, the questions that were asked and the one vital problem that your boss did follow up on — but you did not know which tasks would be important at the time you had to choose how much effort to put into them. Without 20-20 foresight we all have to prepare for the likely eventualities and prioritise our efforts around things that will probably matter, and a few highly unlikely things that would really matter if they did happen — you don't buy car insurance expecting to damage the car, but in case it happens. A lot of other things, like the career that suits our interests or the computer we save up for, rely on the building blocks of the right qualifications or the extra hours of work to save money. Achievement is often said to be 90% perspiration and 10% inspiration, and organisation, selecting priorities and healthy moderation are some of the keys to managing the less enjoyable perspiration.

Inertia is the physical property of an object that resists movement. Some people have a high inertia and take longer to get started on tasks. A simple and practical solution to inertia is, unsurprisingly, exercise. Physical movement and exercise are important in getting the mind working too, and moderate exercise is almost always motivating — there is no such thing as having too little time to spare for exercise. Good diet is also essential to combating inertia and breakfast is the most important meal in starting a productive day — that means fruit or cereal, not just caffeine. Getting into a routine that starts with a light breakfast and exercise will also be a routine that breaks down inertia.

Motivation can be a huge issue for many people. Your interests are simply not aligned with the tasks that face you. It may be that the tasks are essential tasks for making a living, or essential building blocks towards the life that you aspire to, in which case you have to grin and bear the pain. Sometimes you need to seek help — from teachers, employers or the HSE — to find better and less difficult ways of managing the tasks that you need to achieve. Or it may be that your interests and personal satisfaction in life can not be achieved with what you are currently doing, in which case you may need to rethink either your lifestyle or your interests.

Sometimes getting started can seem impossible because you are overwhelmed by complexity and can not see which part of a job needs to be done first, or the whole thing is so complex that it seems like it is impossible. Planning an prioritisation are skills, and they are skills that can be practised and learned. Simply listing the tasks, then breaking down complicated tasks into steps, then ordering the steps into a logical sequence can be all you need to get started. Often just asking the right question is most of the way to finding the right answer.

There is an interesting vacuum between complicated tasks that obviously need a plan (like building an aeroplane) and simple tasks that do not (like finding something to eat). People with autism spectrum disorder may have difficulties with working memory and with sequencing tasks. Working memory is required to juggle a set of details which are just a little too demanding, and just like juggling balls, the effect creates an illusion that there are far more balls in the air than there really are. The simple act of writing a to-do list can alleviate a lot of stress and ensure that tasks get both started and finished, as well as remembered and resumed if they are interrupted.

If you feel that you have no time left after meeting other more urgent demands, then you need to make time by prioritising the demands. Sometimes you will be juggling other people's demands against your own interests, which is always hard. As with the other problems, writing things down can be very helpful, especially when you need to discuss the relative priorities of your interests with somebody who has a demand on your time.

5.1.2 Keeping going

Distractions as a whole and sensory distractions in particular can create a huge mental load and slow you down, stop you on a task or interrupt a task causing extra effort in resuming the task and remembering where you were. Eliminating or reducing sensory distractions can be easy when you control the environment (such as your own home) and many workplaces can accommodate some change when the need is clearly explained. Noise distractions include failing low-energy bulbs that can be changed, clicky keyboards, sound-effects on mobile phones and computers that can be turned down and exterior noises that can be shut out (although this be a compromise with the heat, cold or fresh air). Tactile distractions start with your own clothes, the equipment you sit at (chairs and tables), other surfaces you touch and airflow like breezes. Wearing full-length, natural fabric clothing will protect your skin from unwanted tactile sensations — in fact wearing full-length clothing irrespective of the weather is a tell-tale indicator of autism spectrum disorder, and the 'outdoor' clothes are only taken off in safe home environments. Synthetic, crinkly, rough and sweaty materials can often be changed for others that function exactly the same way, without additional expense. Even pens, keyboards and other equipment can create a tactile distraction that is a continuous and completely unnecessary load on your mind all the time you are attempting to attend to work. Visual distractions include flickering lights (failing tube lights or starters), moving doors, people, reflective surfaces, video or TV displays and the scene outside the window. Some new LED lights can flicker even more intensely than older low energy fluorescent lighting and of course Christmas lighting and decorations are intended to distract. The 3D versions of films can induce a headache or leave you feeling like you have been in a train-wreck. Turning a desk, using a window blind or moving visual distractions to a common area can make a big difference. Odours can often be a sensitive personal subject, especially if it is a colleague's favourite aftershave, snack or post-exercise sweat that is a problem. Other distracting aromas can come from old (especially badly-stored) books and paper, carpet adhesives and synthetic fabrics, as well as any chemicals or foods local to your workspace. Odour is a tough issue to deal with, but ensure that food waste such as banana peel, onion or egg are thrown away elsewhere and not in the area you work in. Taste is something that should not be overlooked because many things related to activity cause taste sensations, including ink, rubbers, paper dust and metals that you taste directly as dust, on your fingers or directly by chewing them (such as pencils). Being aware of the effect of taste sensations, including the after-taste of food and medicine, can make you aware of another distraction that you can deal with.

(It is a constant surprise that many people expect to work, or expect their children to do homework, at the kitchen table surrounded by food smells, breezes, constant motion, the competing sounds of play, radio and television, on furniture at the wrong height — and without any visual reinforcement of the work such as a bookshelf and stationery supplies. This is not, for most people, the best place to work.)

Most external sensations can not be masked with a stronger distraction — an odour-absorbing filter or odour-destroying spray is far more effective than a perfume over a stink. Music will not deal with noise as effectively as reducing the noise, either at source or with in-ear headphone buds or over-ear noise-isolating or noise-cancelling headphones — the headphones do not have to be connected to a music source. Music (and especially rhythmic, dance-style music) is a special case for many people who find that a strong beat, restricted melody and limited vocals can aid concentration and focus. It is as if the rhythmic component of music is entertaining parts of the mind that wander while the rest gets on with work. The most effective musical styles might be electronica, hip-hop, house or rave music that is not particularly pleasurable for relaxation. If music (or indeed aroma or taste) provide a positive sensory engagement with work and a disengagement from distractions, then use it.

Senses that are less often discussed are the vestibular, proprioceptive and interoceptive senses — your awareness of motion and gravitational upright, your sense of your body's locations and your sense of internal feelings. Vestibular sense is important in keeping stimulated and engaged, and vestibular sense is dampened when you are slumped in a poorly-adjusted chair and desk. Some people sit on a special air-cushion or inflated ball that provides continuous vestibular stimulation and requires that you sit upright to avoid falling. Ideally, your feet are both on the floor, your thighs are horizontal, your elbows are level with or slightly above your desk and your eyes are aligned with the centre of the screen or task that you are attending to. Most schools and workplaces have someone trained in ergonomics who can assess the suitability of your own work space, or advise on a home work space. A well-designed work space will also enhance your sense of proprioception, so that movement is more natural and less clumsy, without requiring you to look away and become distracted when reaching for things or changing posture. Interoception is important in ensuring that you notice and respond appropriately to internal feelings, such as needing to use the toilet, becoming stiff from sitting in the same position for too long, or sensations like numbness before they become painful and distracting. Internal senses are always present and mindfulness can help become aware of the nature and location of a sense, so that it is not a nagging distraction.

Executive function difficulties can lead to problems with focus, disorganisation and handling unexpected outcomes or interruptions. To do any task effectively you can ensure that reminders about the task are always to hand, on a noticeboard or in a diary. You may find that you already keep your desk completely clear of everything except the one task you are working on, unlike everyone else you know — another tell-tale sign of an autism spectrum disorder. If you organise your work space, bookcase or toolbox with the things required for the task at hand then those objects can be as good a visual record of the tasks as a to-do list or plan. Keeping an organised work space, where everything has a place and everything is in its place, reduces the mental load of trying to remember vital but distracting details. It may seem like extra effort to always put pencils back in the pencil-pot, needles in the pin-cushion and screwdrivers in the tool-rack, but you always know where to find them if they are in place. It is important to organise the pencil-pot, pin-cushion and tool-rack to be where you reach when you are working and not in the dark cellar, *"on display in the bottom of a locked filing cabinet stuck in a disused lavatory with a sign on the door saying 'Beware of the Leopard'"*, like the public planning notice in Hitchhikers' Guide to the Galaxy.

Some lack of focus, or wandering from the task at hand, can be attributed to hypervigilance and heightened anxiety that are common in people with autism spectrum disorder. It is difficult to switch all your attention to the task if you are uncomfortable, feel unsafe or have nagging thoughts that you can not pin down. Dealing with the distracting thoughts and feelings of safety can create a more productive environment, either by removing features that create anxiety or by creating a less anxious state of mind through prescription drugs, yoga or therapy. The environmental change may be as simple as ensuring that you can see the door instead of working with a door (and the unexpected) behind your back, ensuring that you have sufficient time by agreeing a timetable with other people before starting work, or working at the times when it is quiet and taking breaks when predictable noise occurs.

Keeping the area and materials organised also helps you to switch tasks when disturbed, so that you can answer a doorbell or telephone and then come back to a task that is clearly laid out with visible reminders of what you were doing when you were disturbed. If you use lists of steps or other written instructions, then it helps to cross out or tick the completed steps — and to have the list somewhere that you can see it. Another task-switching problem is in coping with unexpected problems or changes to a plan — perhaps the glue did not work, the encyclopaedia did not contain the information you expected or work-partners did not do their part. In each case your plan has been disrupted and it can feel like it is fatally destroyed by any change to the smooth flow. Often it just takes a break from the job at hand to sit back and reconsider the problem freshly, in exactly the same frame of mind as when creating the initial plan. Of course you are not in the same frame of mind and it appears that something that you are now emotionally invested in has been damaged. However, you are already closer to the desired outcome than you were at the outset and it should be easier to plan forward from this new point, once you have taken a breather.

5.1.3 Moderation

Moderation is all about avoiding a rush-crash cycle of enthusiasm and overwork followed by exhaustion and withdrawal. Once you do get "into the zone" and are completely absorbed in a task that has you totally focused, it can be hard to take breaks or to rest. If a project is particularly stimulating then you might want to work all the way through the night, without eating, until you have finished. You may even feel that this is extremely productive and the way you perform best. It probably is not and you would probably be more effective in the long term if you did take breaks to eat, relax and sleep. Time management is very important — for instance taking a quarter-hour break every couple of hours, not working beyond the normal end of the working day and not spending entire weekends on the same project as you spend the week. Timekeeping is very important. You should always be on time, whether for an appointment or your own schedule, take your breaks in full and set reasonable times to complete tasks, which you can stick to.

Moderation is also about adopting a lifestyle that includes sufficient exercise and a balanced, nutritious diet. A healthy lifestyle includes at least twenty minutes of aerobic exercise (the kind that makes you sweat and your heart pump) three or four times per week, and as much as thirty minutes per day according to some authorities. In any case, it is good to start your day with a light breakfast and some form of physical activity such as a brisk walk or indoor exercise regime. One simple, effective exercise regime that takes no more than 11 minutes per day is the 5BX (Five Basic Exercises) Plan originally developed by the Royal Canadian Air Force, which you can find at en.wikipedia.org/ wiki/ 5BX. Healthy mental function is greatly improved by a basic level of physical fitness, and some moderate physical exercise can kick-start the mind into working better.

Posture, seating and the immediate environment are important to maintaining adequate stimulation without becoming over-stimulated and tired. Slouching on a comfortable sofa surrounded by music and visual distraction is rarely the best place to think or work effectively. Some vestibular stimulation comes from adopting and maintaining an upright posture, and from using suitable furniture to work at. Being physically fit makes it easier to adopt good posture, and to switch between physical and mentally focused, physically inert tasks.

Some mental training can help, if you enjoy or perceive the benefits of the group sessions. Yoga and mindfulness training both develop an awareness of your physical state and the interaction between mind and body. They can both help develop and awareness of how sensations are distracting and create a mental load, which is the first step on the way to eliminating or tolerating those distracting sensations. A sensory diet programme such as skin brushing for tactile defensiveness or auditory integration therapy for hypersensitivity to noise can build a tolerance to previously distracting sensations.

Some drugs affect mental performance, including stimulants like caffeine or Ritalin, anti-anxiety medication and alcohol. Stimulants can help to keep focus on the task that requires attention — an attention-deficient person is usually distracted by attention to all stimuli, whether relevant or not and stimulants can help narrow the focus of attention. Stimulants can also be tiring in the long term because excessive stimulation requires energy and may cause severe exhaustion and social withdrawal later. Anti-anxiety medication can have a similar effect on attention, by suppressing distracting thoughts and reducing the anxiety arising from strange places or unwanted sensations. Anti-anxiety medication also suppresses overall focus and causes drowsiness. Alcohol is a depressant that seems to help you relax, but rarely (especially in excess — and excess is a very small measure) has long term benefits for productivity. Exercise is a cheap method of obtaining some very potent drug effects. Exercise releases the stimulant adrenaline, the pleasure chemical dopamine and the pain-killing feel-good endorphins. They are released in direct proportion to the exercise, in quantities that are usually balanced and not excessive.

5.1.4 Perfectionism

Perfectionism is an excellent driver to get things done well, and often beyond well. Perfectionism becomes a serious problem when the efforts to complete a project perfectly are so demanding that the job is never finished. Often the job is already adequate and possibly already better than anyone requires or expects, but adequate is not good enough for you.

Perfectionism can arise from unrealistic expectations of what you can or what you should achieve. You are unlikely to compose world-class music the first time that you put pen to manuscript paper (or put your mouse to Garage Band), even though you know that Mozart did when he was five. Most achievement takes practice and the road to achievement is full of mistakes. It is very important to accept that many attempts to produce something will fail, and each failure is an opportunity to learn more. Their is a saying that *"if you are not failing, then you are not testing your abilities enough"*.

A great deal of perfectionism arises from a fear of making mistakes and a fear of criticism. Everybody makes mistakes and criticism can be an opportunity to learn. It is important to distinguish positive criticism (where someone is trying to be helpful) from negative and personal criticism. You may often feel that criticism is personal and hurtful even when that was not the intention. The fact that you feel emotional hurt does not mean that the emotional hurt was intended.

Some perfectionism arises from comparison with others and very often this comparison is false. People boast and people lie about their achievements. Everyone from schoolchildren to football stars will exaggerate about how little effort something took to learn or how often they do it. You don't necessarily see the mistakes, and they only remind you about the successes.

5.2 Time and task management techniques

There are many time and task management techniques, some of which are extremely helpful. Some of which are entire personal success programmes (protected by copyright or patent) that are accompanied by training courses, specialised diaries and computer software. Some of these are successfully selling a fantasy without any evidence that their customers learn to be more effective. Most success methodologies rely on similar techniques of making explicit representations out of the implicit requirements to manage time, tasks or resources. Written or visual outcomes are usually different forms of ordered lists and diagrams. These representations free up your working memory to use it for problem solving, they improve executive function and they reduce the stress of managing sequences of tasks.

Some widely-respected personal planning books include David Allen's "Getting Things Done: The Art of Stress-Free Productivity" (2002), Stephen R Covey's "The 7 Habits of Highly Effective People: Powerful Lessons in Personal Change" (2004), Brian Tracy's "Eat That Frog!: 21 Great Ways to Stop Procrastinating and Get More Done in Less Time" (2004) and Mark Forster's "Do It Tomorrow and Other Secrets of Time Management" (2006) — Mark Forster describes his 'autofocus' methodology at lifehacker.com/ 5704856/.

The starting point for problem solving usually starts with questions. The "Five Ws" (What? Where? When? Why? Who?)

and quantity (How much?) will often open up a problem and help you to break it down into separate steps. The steps can then be logically ordered, by how important they are, or by how soon they need completing. Once a first version of the ordered steps has been drafted it may be necessary to review and repeat the process on each of the steps until they are also sufficiently opened up and broken down.

Your outcome might be a list of material resources, a collection of appointments and deadlines or a collection of informational facts and explanations. It might just be a to-do list on the back of an envelope. The process has taken all the thoughts you were juggling, many of which were implicit and poorly-defined, and created a visual reference that is explicit and easy to understand. It is important to ensure that it remains easy to understand by including all the thoughts and facts that you refer to at the time you are writing and might have forgotten by the time you use the plan. For instance "buy book" may become meaningless when you are flustered in a busy bookshop queue, whereas writing the title and author would still be meaningful, and you can hand the paper to the bookshop assistant if you are nervous in shops.

Some typical planning outcomes are shopping lists, to-do lists, schedules, calendar entries, collections of Frequently Asked Questions and essay outlines. Some people like use visual plans such as flowcharts, mind mapping diagrams or project-planning Gantt charts. An alternative planning outcome might be to lay out all the wood, screws and tools into the order that you will need them to build a piece of furniture, or to tidy the kitchen and find all the ingredients to make a cake. Other visual reminders include putting a ring on a different finger to remember an appointment, writing on your hand, putting your keys on your breakfast chair to remind yourself that you need to go somewhere or leaving your lunchbox in the middle of the hallway to be sure to remember to take it when you leave. Sticky-notes are also very good to leave notes on a computer screen or a keyboard, on the television or on the fridge — you are more likely to act on (and then throw away) a note if you stick it somewhere annoying, so that you don't simply collect many disorganised sticky-notes in a pile somewhere without action.

Whatever planning system you use, it should be available to you whenever you need and in the places you need it. One of the simplest, most effective and portable planning systems is a pocket diary and a pencil — if you look at people you work with, people who visit your home, doctors and others with busy schedules, almost all of them will use a diary of some form. Paper and pencil is very reliable (even in the rain and without electricity), but many people prefer a large A4 hardback diary, a wall-calendar in the kitchen, a mobile phone or another solution that contains a diary function of some form. If your day or week repeats, then a timetable is very useful (which is just as true for employees and for parents as it is for school students).

5.2.1 Low technology techniques

Low technology techniques that use pencil and paper have huge advantages that they do not need batteries or chargers, are available everywhere, are easy to synchronize, do not have multiple versions or upgrades, work in the rain and can be read in any light. Most of all, pencil and paper does not require any learning by you or by other people who you discuss tasks with.

A diary or a calendar is one of the most fundamental and universally understood planning tools. Depending on your own needs, you might have a calendar on the wall showing one month on each spread, a diary that fits in your pocket, a bigger book that you can carry in a bag or a desk-diary. The most important factor is that the diary is available whenever (and wherever) you make appointments and whenever you need to be reminded about appointments. If you use a wall-calendar or a desk diary that you leave at home, then it is a good idea to get into the habit of carrying paper and a pencil — a small spiral-bound reporter's notebook is good. A pocket-sized diary, with some space for noting phone numbers or shopping lists, may be sufficient for all your planning. A one-week-to-a-spread diary will show a whole week, from Monday to Sunday, across the left and right sides of the open diary and allow space for more than one appointment on each day. A month-to-a-spread diary (like a wall calendar) may suit you if you have few appointments, whereas a day-to-a-page diary will be necessary if you have many appointments or a lot to write on each day. A diary is automatically sorted into date order, so you are less likely to miss an appointment that you overlooked, or to book two activities into the same time slot. You can buy small (approximately A5 or A6) ring-binders that hold replaceable diaries of different sizes, year-planners, contact details and to-do lists. A ring-binder means that you can insert extra pages into a busy week, replace messy pages and can keep sheets that have contact details or other important information. You can also have some blank sheets at the front or back for disposable shopping and to-do lists.

An ordered list is the basic unit of paper-based planning. A list should have a heading and have a sequential order. It matters more that a list is ordered than what ordering is used — it could be by priority, or by a characteristic like date or alphabetic order. For instance, you could keep your friends' contact details in order of first name, last name or birthday. If an item has a position in the list, then it is easy to find it and it is also easy to check that the item is in the list, and only in the list once. Ordering becomes more important as the list grows, and especially when many documents are kept in a collection. Lists are dynamic things so don't try to avoid changing a list — cross items out when they are not needed, draw arrows when you change the importance of a task, use highlighter pen, underlining or stars to highlight items. Rewrite the list on a fresh sheet of paper when it becomes difficult to read.

Index cards are a very useful tool for handling many kinds of information and they can be sorted in card index boxes. A little stack of blank index cards is easy to keep in your pocket to collect information. An obvious use is to store information like names and addresses in alphabetical order — the cards can be taken out as a reminder that something needs to be done. Index cards can also be used to build up the topics of an essay, and are easy to order and re-order as the essay develops. Individual cards can be rewritten onto new cards you decide to split a topic, or they can be stapled together. The final (tidy and legible) cards can be used as prompts to give a presentation or speech. Cards can also be sorted by date order with repeating and non-repeating tasks under tabs for each month. A card labelled "pay electricity bill" could be dealt with and moved to the next month each time the task comes up. A doctor's appointment can be crossed out or thrown away once complete.

Files hold all kinds of ordered information, whether work-related reference or the detritus of modern life (like old receipts and bills that you might need one day). The type of filing system depends very much on the size of the collection. A plastic bag under the bed is possibly the worst kind of filing system. Ring-binders, concertina files and filing cabinets can hold increasing volumes of paper in sequence. If there are sub-collections of documents that need to be kept in their own order, then plastic pockets can keep them together — for example gas bills in date order, within the paid bills section of a binder.

A much overlooked form of filing that works very well is the shoe-box. If you need to keep receipts, bills or other sheets of paper for future reference (such as filling in a tax form or health insurance claim each year), then you can put each piece of paper in the shoe-box as you receive it. The receipts will be almost perfectly sorted by date at the end of the year, and after you have completed the annual return you can bind and file them somewhere to re-use the empty shoe-box again for the next year.

If you do use to-do lists or some other form of paper to plan your future tasks, then you may also want to store your completed lists as a reference to what you have achieved. Like a shelf-full of home-made jam that you made yourself, your completed lists are a record of achievement. Some people enjoy life-logging where they collect detailed records of everything they do and how long it takes them, like calorie-counting applied to every aspect of life. Some people like to photograph their meals, places they have been and people they have met, no matter how mundane the event seems. (In fact, if you photograph places you find off-putting or frightening, like shopping malls or busy streets, then you may notice details that you miss due to anxiety and become more comfortable when you next go there). Smartphones and other technology can collect more complete life-logs with less effort than paper.

5.2.2 High technology

Technology offers amazing facilities to collect, organise and store information. The most obvious two devices to aid planning are smartphones and either laptop or desktop computers, with a mixture of the bundled applications and additional applications that you choose to install later. The software on a computer usually does more than a smartphone app, but a smartphone fits in your pocket. Technology can become an end in itself, with the pursuit of ever more efficient and comprehensive solutions taking precedence over the problem of planning. Technological solutions should be used when they help, without taking over or becoming a new problem to manage, and some people simply dislike technology.

The Calendar app is one of the most useful features of a smartphone, and worth having even if you rarely or never make voice calls on a mobile phone. A phone calendar can be displayed in many ways, such as forthcoming events, the day, the week or the month, and you can choose a default view that the app will always open with. If you have a Google Mail account or a Microsoft Exchange account, then you can synchronise the Calendar app with an online calendar, and synchronise your computer with the same online calendar. Every appointment that you make with either the smartphone or the computer will appear on the other, and you can check your appointments wherever you have access to a web browser. You will need to add your email account to the Mail app on the smartphone and to use a mail application like Outlook or Thunderbird with a calendar on the computer. Appointments can be set to sound an alarm (or display a silent reminder) before each appointment, and you can set sensible default values, such as an alarm thirty minutes before an appointment, which you can then change for a specific event if you want an earlier alarm or no alarm. There are further features such as sending email or text messages to other people or sharing an online calendar with other people, but you need only use the features that are helpful to you.

The Mail app on a smartphone and email applications like Outlook or Thunderbird allow you to contact people you know, organisations that advertise their email address or fellow students and colleagues. Email applications allow you to add attachments (such as photographs or documents), to contact many people with a single message and to reply using text quoted from a previous message. Mail on a smartphone accesses a server that stores all previous messages, but the phone will only store a limited collection of recent messages — this can be important if you do not have a data connection on the phone. A computer can be set to store every message in an 'offline cache' so that you have access to every message, even without a wi-fi or internet connection, and can search messages for the sender, recipient, any text within the body of the message or the date sent — don't forget to search your 'Sent' box as well as your 'Inbox'. It is important to note that attachments to emails are documents that must have a matching application — the person receiving the file must have the same or a similar application as the sender. A common problem is that documents or presentations saved with the latest version of Microsoft Office can not be read by someone with an older version, and the document needs to be saved again in a version that both people can handle.

Fundamental to calendar and mail applications, as well as text messaging, is the Contacts or People app on a smartphone or the address book within the email application on a computer. The Contacts list stores a name along with one or more telephone numbers, email addresses, physical addresses and other useful information, including free-form notes and an image or photograph. It is simple to select a person by name or image and to then telephone, message or email that person. Their photograph can be set to display when they message or call you, and you can set a different ringtone for each contact. You can synchronise your contacts with a Google Mail or Microsoft Exchange account if you have one, so that contacts are shared with your computer and available anywhere you have access to a web browser.

A plain text editor such as Notepad in Windows, Notes on iPhone or Jota on Android allows you to write reminders, lists or simple notes without any of the distractions of fonts, layout or tables. The smartphone apps will open with the most-recently edited note on display, so if you write a shopping list at home and close Notes or Jota, the list will appear as soon as you open the app in the shop, without having to search for it. In a computer application like Notepad, the File menu displays recently-used file-names. If you keep a To Do list, then you can make it into a perpetual record by adding all new entries at the beginning of the file, typing the date every day or week and moving completed actions under the date. The file represents all your achievements, in reverse date order.

A number of online applications (such as Evernote and Remember the Milk) raise note-taking to a higher level, with synchronisation between phone, computer and online accounts, as well as sharing notes, photographs or events with your calendar and with other people. You can use the features that work for you and ignore the many additional features that you do not find helpful.

There are some useful apps with often overlooked potential on computers and smartphones. The Camera can be used to photograph articles in the newspaper, the television schedule, the settings in a complicated computer application, new clothes you want advice on and all sorts of other visual reminders. You can organise images in the Photos or Gallery app. A computer and digital camera are also useful, although you will need to download the photographs from the camera. The Clock includes a count-down timer and stopwatch that is useful to time an activity, as well as regular alarms for waking in the morning or remembering repeating events, which can be made to ring only on specific days of the week, and with individual alarm sounds. Location and Map apps can not only tell you where you are, they can mark specific locations to visit again, find places by name (including shops and offices) and provide both satellite and street views of the places — these can be incredibly useful ways to view a place before going to it, to have a sense of familiarity with the layout if it makes you more comfortable when going somewhere new. There are also a number of location-aware apps to request Taxis or Minicabs (without making a voice call), which display the locations and likely arrival time of the car. Your own bank may have its own branded app for viewing your bank account and making some transactions by smartphone.

Voice Memos or Voice Recorder allows you to make a recording of your own voice, or any other sound, on a smartphone. You can then listen back, send the recording as a message or email or transfer it to your computer. The quality of the recording should be good enough to record yourself or another person near you who is speaking clearly, in a quiet place. Smartphones are not good for recording in noisy places, or recording distant sounds like a lecturer in a large room. A digital voice recorder, such as those made by Sony, Philips or Olympus, can make good stereo recordings in a variety of locations with sufficient clarity for lectures or meetings. The digital files will typically be named according to the date, assuming that you have set the clock correctly on the recorder, but you can rename and organise them into folders if you transfer them to a computer. A straightforward sound editor such as Audacity or Goldwave will allow you to cut recordings to select the important parts, join pieces together and make more complex adjustments such as changing the volume or reducing background noise. You can use voice recognition software like Dragon Naturally Speaking (or the mobile app Dragon Dictation) to convert clear recordings of a single voice into text that you can subsequently correct and edit.

Data security is very important when you use technological solutions for planning, with three main issues — data loss, portability and privacy. The first and most immediate issue is to create backups (on a memory stick, external hard disk or web storage service) of important data in case your device (phone or laptop) is lost, stolen or damaged. The data from the backup can be restored when you get another device, or read using another device if you need immediate access. It is important to check that you can read your backup data, and to make a backup reasonably often. The second issue is to ensure that your data is portable and transferable, for instance if you buy a new model of phone, or a different version of software or even switch to a completely different operating system. The most important files will be your contacts and calendar (which you will have backed up if you synchronized your contacts and calendar through the internet) and your personal documents, which you should save to a computer in a format that you are sure you will be able to read elsewhere. You can connect by wi-fi (to save on data charges) and email all the important things to yourself if you are stuck. The third issue is your personal privacy and safety — your laptop and phone contain your personal documents and any passwords that you have stored with (for instance) online banking apps, Facebook or other web pages with login details. Most technology thieves have no interest in your personal data, but be aware that anyone who can access your phone or computer will be able to read your email, send email in your name or look at your bank balance. Smartphones can be locked with a PIN or password that is difficult to bypass, but computers can not — it is always possible to boot a computer from a CD-ROM or memory stick to bypass login passwords. You must take reasonable care that you do not lose your device, or leave it unprotected where other people might access it, and especially never leave it logged into your Twitter or email accounts.

5.3 Study and planning activities

Study is a special case of planning that requires all the same solutions as any other problem, and then a few more. Education as we know it, with mass teaching and mass examination, is a relatively new phenomenon — many of the greatest minds in science, from Pythagoras to Newton, were tutored and tested as individuals. Mass schooling became widespread in the nineteenth century, when education was no longer the exclusive privilege of the rich or powerful. Free, universal education is a wonderful benefit, but can constrain non-conformists, such as Thomas Edison ("too stupid to learn") or Albert Einstein ("mentally handicapped"), or people whose abilities are not suited to passing mass examinations. For most of us, unless we are home-schooled, the only two things that matter in the first two decades of education are not getting in trouble with teachers and passing examinations.

Teachers often say that the single most frequent cause of study and exam failure is not reading (or not following) the instructions. It does not matter if you know better methods, more appropriate facts or have brilliant conclusions — they must relate directly to the instructions. The start of all study planning is knowing what is expected of you. This means knowing what topics to learn, what written output is required (in the way of essays, projects or tests), what evidence to produce (such as portfolios and working documents) and how to complete the examination papers. The entire curriculum in Ireland is publicly accessible from the National

Council for Curriculum and Assessment (www.curriculumonline.ie/en/ Post-Primary Curriculum/). Examination materials for past years are available to www.examinations.ie/, providing both the past papers themselves and the marking schemes for assessing them.

Once you know what is required from study, you need to manage the obstacles to getting started (inertia and lack of motivation) whilst limiting the distractions from completing study activities, including excessive focus on the more enjoyable and absorbing parts of study at the expense of the parts that are a chore. Leaving Certificate points are assessed by adding up the scores in your best six subjects (with a bonus for higher level mathematics), so you need to balance your time across the full range of study. One particular issue of concern is that you need to discuss these requirements and your own performance with other people, such as teachers and your parents. These can be uncomfortable discussions, and they often sound like deep personal criticism. They are essential, however, because it is difficult (especially for someone with autism) to have a comprehensive, objective opinion about your own abilities and how they are meeting the requirements of study.

A study environment should be somewhere free of noise and other distractions, with the necessary materials at hand and reminders of study in sight, so that you can immerse yourself in a study zone at the times you devote to study — and, just as importantly for many, leave when you are no longer studying. Moderation is very important and taking breaks helps concentration and aids relaxation.

Perfectionism can be a huge barrier to completing work, and not finishing one piece of work will snowball into not starting others — and, remember, every subject is as important as every other, whatever you feel about the matter. It is important not to obsess about subjects that you value, or to strive for perfection in any one piece of work because you will not be matching your efforts with the priorities imposed by the examination system. Learn what counts and value your own time by achievement — even when you don't agree with the value that others place on it.

In an examination setting, planning is more effective than usual. Read the questions and try to understand what they are asking, and how they relate to the curriculum. Not answering the question (or answering a question that is not the one printed in the examination paper) is one of the most frequent reasons for exam failure. Take time at the beginning of the exam session — perhaps 15% (that is 10 minutes per hour of exam) — to study the paper, note the topics addressed and the possible solutions. You might want to have a single side of paper to write some notes during this planning phase, to decide which questions to answer if there is any choice, or what direction you might pursue in essay answers. Schedule the time and divide it equally according to the marking scheme — don't spend time on the parts you know and love at the expense of marks elsewhere. Keep moving through your schedule so that you complete the whole paper, and do not spend too much time on questions that you are struggling with. In most examinations you are free to answer the questions in any order, so it makes a lot of sense to complete the easy questions first, before starting the ones that you expect to have difficulty with. If you are able to schedule some time to check over answers, then do so. If managing anxiety and maintaining a positive mood are an issue, then it can help to be sure that you have dressed comfortably, that you are not too hot or too cold and that you have a bottle of water with you. A personal item like a cuddly toy or a holiday souvenir that makes you feel happy or secure can be helpful, either on the desk in sight or inside a pocket.

5.4 Planning travel and events with other people

Travel plans are a special case where prior knowledge and shared expectations can make an experience more enjoyable and productive for everybody concerned. Planning is helpful whether you are going to travel alone, with family or friends, or with work colleagues. Some of this section applies equally well to **any** event where details like timing and the presence of other people might cause you concern — even common events like Christmas dinner or a night in with friends can work better if the details are known beforehand. A lot of people are happy to go along with the flow of events as they unfold, spending their time with whoever happens to show up — some people even take an unscheduled flight to a foreign country carrying only a backpack to see what will happen (and they enjoy doing it). This, to me personally, is a terrifying prospect — I need the security of knowing precise details in advance. It is easier to accept that plans might change than to have no plan and worry constantly when I could relax. I can even manage to do things spontaneously, if I have the safety net of a plan to fall back on if I feel the plan would work better.

Concrete details help. I have difficulty when people say we will do something "later", "sometime" or "we will definitely get around to it" (when?!), because I need concrete details. It is much easier if someone makes an educated guess that "we will arrive at 10" — assuming the traffic is as good as usual and we travel at the usual speed. It is not helpful to introduce unnecessary worries like "if there isn't a fatal multiple-vehicle collision on the motorway" or "as long as the plane doesn't catch fire", **unless** this is a shared style of humour that helps everyone defuse tension about travelling.

A simple illustration of the importance of precise information is the popularity of weather forecasts or horoscopes — they are inaccurate, but they convey a sense of precision in a world that is subject to change. The forecast is only guide that is often wrong in detail, but it helps you to form a plan. I even use an internet site with hour-by-hour rainfall forecasts to decide when to go out of the house, because it is helpful to have concrete plans, even knowing that the forecast is made with uncertain information that is going to change. I sometimes get wet, but at least I have a plan and follow it through, instead of sitting at home anxiously waiting for dry weather, and arguing with other people about when the sun might come out.

5.4.1 Security restrictions when travelling

Since the 9/11 terrorist attacks in the US, airports and travel terminals all over the world have a heightened sense of security that is intimidating. It will smooth your passage though check-in and security if you have everything you need and follow the advice of the airline on what items you may and may not carry. You should pack a single carry-on bag that contains everything you will need on the flight or journey, within the permitted carry-on weight.

Some airlines require that hold luggage is pre-booked and will charge an excess fee if you arrive at check-in with luggage that has not been pre-booked, or if it exceeds the weight allowance. You must not carry any of the prohibited items, which vary between travel operators and travel terminals. You will need relevant travel documents — proof of travel, identity documents, proof of relationships and evidence of any disability — in a zipped-up pocket of your carry-on luggage, a neck-strap or a secure pocket. Proof of travel may be printed at home with some airlines, and may be exchanged for another document (e.g. a boarding card) at check-in. Many travel terminals have websites with maps and guides to navigating between terminals or through check-in and security, which you can study beforehand or print and bring with you.

If you travel with medication or have any form of implant, then you should carry evidence such as a prescription form, pharmacy dispensing docket or a letter from your doctor. You may wish to travel with a letter explaining any behaviours that you know the travel staff might find unusual — for instance any nervous ticks, extreme nervousness or the possibility of a sensory meltdown. A card or letter stating that you have a diagnosis on the autism spectrum can be helpful in these instances. It is not possible to travel with large bottles of liquid, and many flights no longer serve any form of free drinks. The current limit at Irish airports is 100 ml, and it is possible to buy travel containers of this size at pharmacies which you could use if you need a small amount of water to swallow medication on a flight.

It is a good idea to keep all your documents such as the boarding card, even when you complete the flight. Some airports insist on seeing a boarding card as evidence for connecting flights. Even if you do not understand or agree with security procedures, it is best to be prepared and not to question authority.

Security procedures now have a big sensory and emotional impact, especially for people with sensory issues or anxiety. Security personnel are highly visible and carry large weapons. The 'pat-downs' are much more frequent and may include feeling around your thighs or running fingers around the inside of your waist-band. They may ask you to remove your jacket, belt and shoes, and to pass through the scanner more than once (if you forgot to remove keys from your pocket). Security checks will be easier if you carry fewer items and wear simple clothing — you can put your watch, phone, mp3-player and headphones into your carry-on bag before the search.

5.4.2 The basics of planning travel and events

The 'five Ws' are fundamental questions that help anticipate uncertainty — **What** are we going to be doing? **Who** is going to be there? **When** is this happening? (or more completely: when will it start, how long will it last, and when will it end?) **Where** are we going to be? **Why** are we doing it?

Agree a plan. Make out a plan with as little or as much detail as everyone involved needs and agree the plan with everyone else. Your plan can use precise times, based on reasonable travel times and stays at each point. Guide books (like The Rough Guide or Lonely Planet) are a mine of useful, detailed information about routes, opening times and even the food available almost anywhere on Earth. Take a look at the guide to Ireland and your home area for an idea of how comprehensive and useful these series can be. There are plenty of specialist guides to restaurants, museums, hotels and hostels in most bookshops, and a treasure-trove of information on the internet. Many internet sites will contain photographs of places (all the way from the airport to the hotel, via photographs of each bus and train service, if that happens to soothe your anxieties) that you could print and put into a folder as your own timetable guide.

Expect change. A plan is not the future, just a guide to a set of opportunities. Sometimes plans do unfold exactly as expected (in fact many people get quite angry if other people turn up late for work, miss meetings or drag appointments out into the lunch-break) and sometimes they change. No plan is perfect and often there will be many different plans that are equally good and all of which offer the same set of opportunities — you could easily rearrange the order in which you visit Disneyland attractions, and might well do so in response to the different lengths of queues or how tired members of your group are.

Be reasonable. Few plans will unfold exactly as expected, unexpected opportunities may be better than the things you had planned and people change their minds. Trying to stick rigidly to a plan when everyone else wants to do something different or when circumstances change is a recipe for conflict and anxiety. Be reasonable about changes, but also expect others to be reasonable when you explain why order and expectation are important to you — and, of course, be sure that you do share these personal needs. It is also important to be reasonable with the people you meet while travelling, especially people in official positions — uniformed security staff may want to search you, museum staff may tell you that an exhibit is closed to the public, guides may request that you follow an approved route. There is no point telling them that their rules conflict with your plans, because you will lose the argument. Sometimes it can be very helpful to tell officials that you have an autism spectrum disorder, or even to show them an ID card or autism alert leaflet explaining what autism is — especially if you are upset and feel like you might have a meltdown because they are unreasonably destroying your plan. You still won't win any arguments, but most officials will be much more reasonable and informative in explaining their rules and suggesting alternative ways of handling the situation.

5.4.3 How planning helps

Planning reduces anxiety. Planning the What, Who, When, Where and Why of events helps to provide a collection of prior knowledge of what to anticipate in an outing or event, knowing who else will be there and how long they will be there for. This knowledge reduces anxiety caused by ruminating about unknowns — events might unfold differently and the people involved might choose or be forced to change the plans, for instance if a museum is unexpectedly closed.

Planning reduces conflict. If everyone involved has a shared expectation of what they are doing, they can enjoy the experience more without discovering that they all have different plans, different expectations or different interests.

Planning maximises opportunities. This is true whether you are planning a get-together at home or a complicated trip to tourist sites in a foreign city. Knowing the list of places that you all wish to visit or the list of activities, along with all of their usual opening times and costs, will allow the group to create a day-by-day (or hour-by-hour) timetable of planned events. Some of these might be 'must-do' priorities, while others might be desirable but not essential. The plan can be seen as a mosaic of tiles that can be slid around or interchanged if necessary. Some people who cope well with uncertainty and spontaneity might think this planning is a kill-joy pursuit of efficiency over pleasure. If you thrive on certainty, then it is important to express why planning is helpful to you, how much more you enjoy yourself when you know plans in advance and to have a shared agreement about how flexible each person can be.

5.5 Summary

This chapter has presented a lot of material, and if we were to distil it down to a few tips for effective management of your time and resources, then these are some suggestions:

- Make plans, even for insignificant things
- Divide tasks down into steps, and keep dividing the steps
- Keep clear, consistent notes of your plans
- Always be on time
- Create routine wherever it is appropriate
- Don't peck at tasks, finish something
- Create and maintain an environment for getting things done
- Persist when things are hard and when you make mistakes
- Expect mistakes, even in good work — don't get hung up on perfection
- Agree expectations with others when it matters

You should pick whatever works for you, try the ones that look promising and ignore whatever does not help you.

6 Activities of daily living
(Diarmuid Heffernan)

This chapter will look at ways you can organise your everyday life which may make it less stressful and more routine to you. Many people with ASDs have poor organisational skills but being organised around everyday activities can be reassuring, it can reduce anxiety and it can make living with others (or being lived with!) a more enjoyable experience. Many people with an ASD may find social situations difficult and this in turn may effect your ability to communicate with housemates/co-habitors and thus increase potential tensions. The ability of people with an ASD to plan and be organised may also be effected by issues such as feeling overwhelmed and having a 'meltdown' when faced with situations which make you anxious, losing track of priorities because of being engrossed in obsessive interests, or adhering too strictly to routine which may exclude the possibility of change. Lastly, the difficulties many people with an ASD may face in terms of tidiness and organisation may be because of leaving the family home without having learned these practical skills.

6.1 Tidiness and organisation

Being tidy can have a positive effect on you and on the people you may share with. Very often, arguments occur between those in shared accommodation because of untidiness or lack of cleanliness. In terms of tidiness it is important that you play your part in keeping shared areas of a house tidy. Using a roster to decide who does what and when is often a good way of everyone contributing and it diminishes the potential flashpoints for argument. If you are living alone then keeping your space tidy is also important in terms of your positive mental health. It is often difficult to begin to tidy somewhere if you have lived there for a number of months or years and have not attempted to tidy, so it is best to create positive tidying and cleanliness routines from the time you move in somewhere as otherwise clutter can quickly build up and begin to dominate your space.

A fundamental part of being tidy is being organised. There are a variety of reasons why people with ASDs may have difficulties with organisational skills such as limitations in social skills which may make the idea of dealing with others including public servants, housemates etc very difficult. Difficulties with working memory, getting too engrossed with particular topics of interest to the detriment of other important issues such as answering mail/keeping living space clean etc. For many people with an ASD the need for routine may lead to difficulties in responding to unexpected changes or interruptions and this may create conflict with housemates. An example of this may be a house-share where the various housemates clean/tidy/cook in an ad hoc way rather than adhering to a rota. In this instance it may be advisable to try and fit in with the routine if it is possible for you to do so, maybe you could propose doing a specific task every day or week or you could explain politely that you prefer a rota system as it is clear and easy to follow.

In general a very good first step in being organised is to purchase a diary in which you can write the tasks you need to do each day. This may include letters to reply to, work tasks, tidying your abode, walking the dog, sending birthday cards etc (You may also use a PC-based calendar as suggested in chapter 5). It is also worth purchasing a number of folders in which you can place different pieces of paperwork that are necessary to keep. For instance, you may have a folder with all your bank statements and correspondence in it, you may have one with all your utility bills, one with your correspondence with work, the Welfare Department etc. Though much of this type of correspondence is also sent online, most official correspondence also has a physical copy and it is good practice to keep this in case you need to follow a paper trail. It is also important to respond to e-mails, letters and phone calls from official/Government/work etc sources as they may involve issues around, for example, your Social Welfare payments, changes to your utility bills or arrears. Though it may be difficult and stressful to deal with these correspondents, it ultimately creates more anxiety to ignore them. It is good practice if you categorise your correspondence into folders and reply one by one. Try not to feel overwhelmed if there a number to reply to, break them down into single responses and deal with them systematically. If you have been contacted online the same rules apply, set aside some to reply and go through each systematically.

6.2 Cleaning

There are many interesting paradoxes around cleanliness, tidiness and hygiene for people with an ASD. The paradox of not cleaning yet being germ phobic is a relatively common one for people with an ASD. For many people with ASDs the sensation of touching certain materials or the possibility of touching something with germs can be overwhelming. A practical way of overcoming difficulties around handling cleaning products or touching things which may have germs is by using latex or rubber gloves. If you have sensory issues around the wearing of latex or rubber gloves it may be best to seek alternative methods/materials and to wash hands before and after, washing your hands with anti-bacterial soap or an alcohol based hand sanitizer.

It is important to keep the space you live in comfortable for you and for those you may share with. Part of doing so involves cleaning. This includes washing and drying your dishes and putting them away. Find a washing up liquid that works best and make sure it does not irritate your skin, this will be done by trial and error or by exposing a small sample area of your skin to the product before using it. If you have a dishwasher then its best to use good quality dishwasher tablets, there are many on the market now that are also eco-friendly. It is important to clear food from crockery and cutlery before putting them into the dishwasher as this may clog the filter. It is also important to clean the dishwasher with dishwasher salts on roughly a monthly basis. Cleaning the shower or bath regularly with bleach or bathroom cleaning spray is also advisable. Similarly it is best to use products that do not irritate your skin if they come in contact with it. If you are still worried about this then it may be worthwhile purchasing rubber/latex gloves to protect your skin. The toilet also needs to be cleaned regularly and as necessary, there are many products that serve this purpose such as bleach, however there are also many eco-friendly products which work equally well, or indeed the trusty toilet brush and some elbow grease! Find a sweeping brush and mop that are efficient and durable for sweeping and washing floors (this may sound obvious but many supermarkets for example, sell low priced goods that are not durable, sometimes it is worth making the effort and paying a little more for something that will last longer and do a better job). Carpets should be vacuumed regularly, there are many options in terms of vacuum cleaners but our advice would be to look at online reviews of products prior to purchasing them. Skirting boards should be cleaned regularly using a sweeping brush or a damp cloth (a potential easier and more efficient way of doing this is to wrap a damp cloth around the head of a sweeping brush and brush the skirting board with it — just remember to clean the cloth at regular intervals). Bed clothes should be washed frequently, and it is important to find a washing powder or washing gel that does not cause any skin irritation for you. Towels, dish towels etc should also be washed regularly. It is useful to purchase a laundry basket and to try and wash as you go — in other words try to keep the laundry basket empty rather than always overflowing with garments etc to be washed! Keeping your living space clean not only may maintain or improve your relationship with those you share with but is also more healthy and hygienic. Not cleaning may also cause difficulties with your landlady or landlord if you are in rented accommodation, and in extreme cases may even lead to conflict and argument.

6.3 Clothing

As stated in chapter four of this book it is important to find clothes that you are comfortable with. This may mean finding fabrics that do not irritate your skin such as natural cotton or wool in preference to synthetic fabrics. Many people also remove all the tags from clothes (including me!) because they are irritating. It is important to have appropriate clothes for appropriate occasions and indeed for different seasons. Many people organise their wardrobe in order of season, with, for example, winter clothes kept separately from summer clothes, or out of season clothes etc. Whether you decide to organise your clothes in this way or not it is worth remembering that wearing a heavy winter coat on a hot summers day may cause some stares from the general population though probably not other people with ASDs!. More important is that you wear appropriate clothes for appropriate occasions, a job interview may be one example where you may need to wear more formal wear such as shoes, tie etc.

For women, it is important to dress in what you are comfortable with, but differs slightly from men, in that, women are subjected to more attention and comment, both positive and negative (please note, we are not trying to prescriptively tell anyone what to wear — male or female — rather we are pointing out the potential reactions based on different style choices) depending on what you choose to wear.

When purchasing clothes it is worth seeking out shops that you are relatively comfortable shopping in. When looking for such shops it is worth taking into consideration factors such as whether the shop is located in a busy area/street, what times or days the shop may be less busy (generally clothes shops will be busier at weekends), if there are sensory factors such as loud music playing or fluorescent lighting in the shop which may have sensory implications for you. It is also worth finding a shop where you are relatively comfortable interacting with the staff of the shop, for example many people are happy to browse a clothes shop until they find clothes they are interested in, while others prefer more advice or help from shop staff. The way of finding a shop you are more comfortable in is through trial and error. If you cannot find a shop you feel comfortable in or cannot find clothes you are comfortable in then it may be worth seeking clothes online. There are a huge variety of options for clothes bought online now but it is worth being aware that sizing may be variable in different countries or indeed with different labels (in my experience a 'large' size in one label/brand may differ greatly in size from a 'large' size in another label/brand). Try to use reputable sites and there may be some trial and error involved in finding suitable sizes/styles/materials, it is best to use a site that gives you a money-back option if you return the garment. It is also common for people with ASDs to buy two or more of the same item of clothing if they fit well and are comfortable.

Many people now want to shop ethically. This can be a tricky proposition given the amount of clothes that are produced in 'sweat shops' in many parts of the world. It is often worth doing some online research into the means and whereabouts of the manufacture of clothes before you purchase them. If it is not possible to buy ethically produced clothing due to finances (as ethically produced clothes are often more expensive) or lack of suitable clothes, then there are charity shops in most cities and many small towns, many of which sell good quality recycled clothes (either new or second hand and many are branded fashion labels), and your purchase price goods towards good causes (I admit a bias towards clothes bought in charity shops as most of my wardrobe consists of clothes purchased in this way!).

6.4 Managing a wardrobe

It is important for many people with an ASD that they 'manage' their wardrobe. Most people have never been given any pointers as to how to do so and there is an implicit assumption that everyone will just know how to without ever being shown. We suggest that there are some practical ways to manage your wardrobe which will make this a relatively straightforward task. For example, being sure that you have everything you need in terms of weather and context appropriate clothing. It is important for example to have at least one formal outfit for interviews etc (e.g. a suit). It is good practice to put out of season clothes away to make space and while doing so it may also be an opportunity to sort out the clothes you never wear. For example if you hang all clean shirts to the right of the wardrobe then unworn items will migrate to the left. You could then take the things you never wear, and are never likely to wear, to a charity shop or give them away to friends/family.

Most important in terms of clothes is that you wash and dry them as you wear them. Read labels on clothes and follow instructions regarding temperatures clothes should be washed and dried at (something I have failed to do on many occasions — to the detriment of my clothes!) for instance tumble-drying a woollen garment will make it shrink. Most modern washing machines have an eco-option which allows for clothes to be washed at low temperatures — generally 30-40 degrees. This is a good general option as it is both environmentally friendly and means less wear and tear on clothes. For specific types of fabric such as wool or silk, it is best to consult the label and follow the instructions. Many garments suggest a hand-wash. It is useful to have a plastic bowl for this purpose, use lukewarm to warm water with some washing powder or gel to wash the garments. If the product could potentially irritate your skin then use latex or rubber gloves to protect yourself. You can leave the clothes to soak for a minimum of an hour before emptying the bowl and removing excess water from the garment. In general these types of fabric need to be dried on a clothes line outside if you have the space for one where you live, or a clothes horse near a window or a radiator etc (please note it is not advisable to put clothes too near, or indeed draped over, sources of heat as this may create a fire hazard). When washing clothes by machine or by hand it is best to try and wash similar colours together as much as possible. For example you may not have a full wash worth of reds but it is advisable not to wash reds and whites together as colours bleed from all dyed fabrics. It is best to wash similar colours together. There are products that 'soak up' the colours that run in a wash but we cannot verify these claims. If ironing clothes, follow the manufacturers guidelines regarding temperatures to iron clothes at.

If you have a tumble/condenser dryer, make sure to check the labels on your garments etc to ensure they can be dried in this way. The use of a clothes dryer is a time efficient way of drying your clothes but is generally not energy efficient, it also serves to lead to a shorter life span for clothes. It is also extremely important to clean the filters in the dryer as the build-up of lint in the filter can create a fire hazard.

If you do not have a washing machine or dryer or cannot use them for whatever reason, you may need to use a laundrette. This is a relatively expensive option and the more clothes needing to be laundered the more expensive it is. It is worth noting that while laundrettes generally do a good job, they may not be as meticulous in checking labels for washing instructions as you are, therefore be selective in the clothes you get laundered and if you can hand wash something yourself rather than laundering it, then it may be wise to do so.

Finally, some clothes need dry cleaning rather than being washed. There are many dry cleaners dotted around cities and many towns in Ireland. Check the label on your garments and if they need to be dry cleaned then check the nearest/most competitive dry cleaners to you either online or through the yellow pages section of your telephone directory.

6.5 Self care and cleanliness

Self-care and cleanliness may seem obvious to some people but may be an issue for others. Most people with an ASD have sensory issues and this may have an impact on their hygiene. There are a number of reasons for this. For example, for some it is the feeling of soap on their skin or even just being wet, for others it is not a priority and for others again it may be because of difficulties in planning or routine. There are ways you can offset these issues (if they apply to you), for example, using brushes/sponges/hand-cloths to wash, minimising time feeling wet by stepping under the shower initially until your body is wet and then stepping back from under the direct stream of water to lather up and wash, then stepping back under to rinse off.

The best way of creating a routine is by gradually building it into your life using set times/days as appropriate. This means, for instance, showering and/or bathing at least once a day (or more often depending on whether you are doing physical work or how much you perspire). The purpose of this is both for hygiene reasons for yourself as an individual and also because not bathing may lead to reactions to body odours which can cause embarrassment in social situations. It is good practice to bathe even on the days you may not be meeting anyone as it promotes positive self esteem. If you do find certain soaps etc harsh to your skin then seek out 'unscented', 'lanolin free' or 'hypoallergenic' products, which you may find less irritating to the skin.

Integral to self care is dental hygiene. Many people with ASDs neglect their teeth either for reasons of lack of self esteem or because they dislike the sensations of toothpaste and/or brushing. Oral hygiene, however is more than just an aesthetic exercise. Oral or dental infections, if left unattended may become quite serious as they can potentially lead to infections, as well as being associated with heart disease and stomach ulcers. Milder medical complications may also accompany many dental infections. These include bad breath, gingivitis, gum disease, fever, general ill feeling, elevated body temperature and swollen lymph glands.

Therefore it is very important to find a toothpaste and a type of toothbrush that you are comfortable with (for example the rotary or ultrasonic toothbrush manufactured by many different companies requires less friction in terms of brushing and thus may cause less discomfort). It is also very important to visit a dentist on a regular basis, every six months is a reasonable visit rate unless you have dental or oral issues such as toothache, painful gums, a chipped or cracked tooth etc, that need to be examined sooner.

6.6 Cooking, eating and kitchen cleaning

Whether you live alone or share your lived space with others, cooking for yourself is a fundamental skill. You do not have to be a master chef, rather it is important to be able to cook sufficient amounts of healthy food (a varied and balanced diet is essential to good health) — proficiently enough to be able to enjoy it. This takes practice and patience. While for some it comes more naturally, for others it requires patience and repetition to get it right. If you are starting to learn how to cook it may be worthwhile investing in a simple cookbook with recipes which are easy to cook and healthy. Alternatively, you can go online and pick up recipes from sites such as www.cookbooks.com/ or www.recipes.com/ amongst many others.

When choosing what to cook it is best to look at what is healthy to eat rather than just what is easy to cook. For instance, frying sausages for dinner every day may be easy but would not constitute a healthy balanced diet! An example of a nutritious, healthy meal which is relatively quick and easy to make may be a stir fry or indeed a salad. Many people with ASDs prefer to eat plain food and may have a tendency to always eat the same food rather than trying new food types or ways of cooking. If this sounds like you, try to expand your palette, not just for the adventure of trying new foods but also to have a balance in your diet which is necessary for good health. There are different ways of having a healthy diet or ingesting healthy food. For instance, if you do not like eating fruit as it feels uncomfortable in your mouth, then it may be worth purchasing a blender or juice extractor so that the fruit juice can be drunk rather than the fruit being eaten. There are also other options for including fruit and/or vegetables in your diet such as dried fruit pieces, fruit in cereals, yoghurts, or soups.

If you are cooking in a shared kitchen, it is generally expected that you would wash, dry and put away any utensils, pots, pans or dishes you have used. It is often wise to have a cleaning roster in a kitchen in shared accommodation regardless of whether it is your family home or not. This prevents potential flashpoints around the performance of domestic duties. Apart from washing up after yourself it is best to clean your oven and fridge whenever they are dirty and at least once a month (depending on use) and to sweep and mop the floor very regularly.

It may also be worth having a shared cooking rota, in this way there would be less work for everyone, more variety in terms of different foods or different methods of cooking.

6.6.1 Shopping for food

In this section we will concentrate on the practical aspects of food shopping. When going food shopping it is a good idea to write a shopping list. Base this on what foods you need (and can afford), having done an inventory of what food you already have in your abode (if you keep food in storage jars or boxes it is easy to see what it is). It is advisable for overall health to try and purchase healthy foods as these are often the easiest to make as well — for example salads. Most supermarkets are generally laid out in a similar fashion now, with confectionery generally inside the door when you arrive before you get to the food-stuffs. Depending on the time of day you shop at and the day of the week, there is usually reduced foodstuff which is about to go out of date. This food is often a good value way of purchasing nutritious food at a reasonable price. The 'Best Before' date is often a guideline and is a way of protecting the manufacturer of the food from claims against them. We are not advocating eating foods which are weeks or months beyond their best before date! We are merely saying this is a guideline rather than a rule, for example, if you have a packet of Crackers a day past its best before date it may still be fine — the easy way to check if food is still viable is to smell it, (Please note you should never use food after its 'Use By' date). If in doubt look up www.safefood.eu/.

Try to keep food waste to a minimum as it is not economical and may cost you more in terms of bin charges if you are binning a lot of food. A good way of having sufficient food is to stock up on non-perishable food such as canned foods — (beans, tuna, chickpeas etc), or to purchase frozen foods (if you have enough freezer space — though you could consider buying a separate freezer/freezer box if necessary). Frozen foods generally have a longer shelf life than non frozen food. Buying frozen food (or buying food that can be frozen) may also allow you to manage your food more efficiently and cut down on waste. Frozen vegetables retain the health benefits of fresh vegetables, yet have a much longer 'shelf life' and are an example of a foodstuff that can be managed more efficiently when frozen. Try to use up the food in your freezer rather than stockpiling as frozen food does have an expiry date also (although generally much longer than fresh fruit).

6.6.2 Catering for a group

Most people, as part of college life, adulthood etc, will be expected to cook for others. This is often as a return favour for having others cook for you and is generally a tacit expectation that if others have cooked for you, that you will return the hospitality and cook for them. Cooking for others is also a way of generating social interaction, or to put it another way cooking for and eating with, groups is generally not just a functional way of slaking an appetite, it is also a way of creating social interaction.

Cooking for a group is a task that involves cooking skill, timing and organisational skills. If you have decided to undertake this task then it is best to begin with a plan. Firstly confirm how many people you are catering for (you might do this by text, e-mail, phonecall etc) and also check to ensure none of your guests have food allergies, whether they are vegetarian, vegan, fruitarian, whether their religious beliefs mean they cannot eat certain foods, or eat certain foods at certain times or whether they are not partial to particular foods. It might be worth checking with your guests what drink they prefer (e.g red wine, white wine, beer, fruit juice etc) or whether they drink alcohol or not. Next it is wise to write a menu base on the information you have been given and on what foods are accessible to you. Then write a shopping list based on the menu and purchase the food.

When planning the timing of your meal, look at the cooking times of each course — it may become stressful if the starter takes longer to cook and consequently comes out after the main course! Therefore it may be worth planning your starter or a first course that can be prepared in advance, possibly even the day before. Choose courses which can be kept hot whilst everything else is being readied, and organise cutlery and crockery before preparing the food.

Using a timer is often a way of keeping your cooking on track and if it is possible to do some preparation of the meals during the day before the arrival of any guests then this may make the cooking a little easier. Try to wash utensils and put things away as you cook as this way your kitchen does not become too cluttered. If you are starting to feel overwhelmed it might be worth enlisting the help of someone else rather than to risk getting overly stressed. Most importantly of all, if you decide to cook for guests, try to enjoy yourself — being host and enjoying the experience should not be mutually exclusive!

7 Non-Asperger syndrome medical issues (Stuart Neilson)

In this chapter we discuss a range of medical and health issues that are not directly related to autism spectrum disorder. Everyone has health issues throughout life and the vast majority will have contact with various health and medical professionals. There is also an increasing trend to medicalise more and more issues that would previously have been seen as within the bounds of normal experience — there is debate about the benefits of turning normal experience into 'problems' and finding medical solutions to those new problems. For instance, the new DSM-5 allows low mood following bereavement to be classified as a depressive episode and treated with drugs, which some people may think a great benefit and others may think interferes with the reality of human experience.

While this chapter is about medical and health issues that are not directly related to autism spectrum disorder, you may have found a strong relationship between many health issues and autism in your own life — there is a strong interaction between feeling unwell and emotional or sensory issues, illness may disrupt your life more than it disrupts other people's lives (especially in relation to your needs for routine and continuity) and you will often see some of the same health professionals in relation to both sets of issues. It is really worth emphasizing that not every health issue in the life of someone with autism spectrum disorder is **not** part of autism, no matter how related they seem or feel, and that the treatment for medical issues will be the same, except with some added sensitivity to your individual nature. It is also worth emphasizing that we are all individuals and that your own individual differences and sensitivities are not all caused by autism — every person is a unique individual, with their unique variations.

There can be a particular problem, and a potentially harmful problem, of identifying everything as autism-related and missing real medical issues in their early stages — and medical professionals are as guilty as anyone in this. You feel unwell or distressed and dismiss it as one of your "bad autistic days", or go to your doctor who dismisses it as another symptom of autism. A few days or weeks later, after more bad days, you are diagnosed with a viral infection or being assessed for a mood disorder. A good judgement call of whether something is a medical problem is whether the symptoms and feelings are **new to you**, and a change from the way you normally feel. No matter what you or a doctor may say about something being "a bit autistic", if there is change then it is quite possibly not a part of your autism, which is relatively stable across a lifetime. You might have bad days, and changes in your contact with other people or your circumstances might exacerbate your existing symptoms, but autism symptoms will not get significantly better or worse from month-to-month.

7.1 The health system in Ireland

The health system in Ireland is a unique mixture of public and private services, with a pervasive historical element of religious patronage — many hospitals were built and operated by the church as charitable enterprises, and have been assimilated into the general health service. The Health Service Executive was recently — in 2005 — established to centralise the administration of regional health boards and to provide a single public agency overseeing services like the Drug Payment Scheme and access to emergency and specialist care.

7.1.1 The general practitioner (GP)

Most people will initially access health care through their family doctor, also called a general practitioner (GP). The general practitioner will assess and treat most medical conditions, which includes requesting all necessary diagnostic tests (like blood samples or X-rays) and prescribing drugs or other therapy. The general practitioner may refer some conditions on to a specialist (a consultant doctor in a medical speciality) for further assessment when it is serious, when it requires special training or when it requires access to special equipment — anything from unusual skin complaints, through infections that are not the usual cold or flu to potentially serious conditions like growths or bleeding that might indicate a cancer. Being referred to a specialist does not mean that something serious is wrong with you, but may mean that the doctor has spotted something that needs to be looked at, or that might become serious if left untreated. We also have great admiration for doctors who admit that they do not know something, rather than trying to portray an image of knowing everything — so we respect doctors who admit ignorance on a specific issue and take out a reference book, phone a consultant are ask the practice nurse for a professional opinion.

You will have to pay for each general practitioner appointment, usually about €50 (but doctors can set their own fees, so it varies from place to place). Most out-of-hours treatment is handled by a locum service that may have access to your records, but is staffed by different doctors. Home visits are not common, but might be arranged if you are too sick to get out of bed or feeling so emotionally unstable that aggression or self-harm is likely. Out-of-hours consultations and home visits cost more. You should consider calling an ambulance if there is a serious risk of injury or death (for instance if someone has stopped breathing, or has taken an overdose of drugs).

General practitioners are also the first place to ask for routine treatments that are part of life. Many people will see their general practitioner for advice about contraception, fertility and family planning advice — and questions about sex, such as painful intercourse or other difficulties with having sex. People ask their general practitioner about any changes to their health or regularity, especially if their is pain, discomfort or inconvenience — all of these are ill-health, even when they are not a disease, and a doctor may be able to help. Some examples include any change to bladder or bowel habits (incontinence, or frequent constipation or diarrhoea), any form of bleeding that is not normal menstrual bleeding (such as blood in your urine or stools), difficulty swallowing or digesting food (including heartburn and reflux of stomach acid into your throat) and any form of itching, skin discolouration, rashes or abnormal discharge of fluids (which might indicate an infection). Some of these issues — especially in relation to sexuality — have a personal element that requires trust between you and your doctor, as well as the confidence that your privacy will be respected, especially if you have the same doctor as your partner or your parents. If you have any doubt about your emotional safety, then ask the doctor to confirm issues about confidentiality or their attitudes to the subject before your reveal personal details. Some doctors (like anyone else) simply have old-fashioned, religious or opinionated views about topics like contraception and sexual orientation. If you still feel unsafe, then seek another care provider — there are family planning and sexual health clinics in most cities. Find the general practitioner who is right for you, by asking other people you know or even your current general practitioner.

Emotional difficulties like anxiety or feeling unhappy are also something you can discuss with a general practitioner. Everyone feels moments of anxiety and low mood, but it is a health issue if you have anxiety that prevents you from completing normal activities of daily living, if you have panic attacks that make you leave places like busy shops or if you have a low mood that extends for more than a few weeks. If you have a low mood that is also accompanied by feeling worthless, not enjoying activities that you would normally enjoy and having thoughts about harming or killing yourself, then there is a possibility that you are experiencing depression. Anxiety and depression are both treatable with counselling and with prescription drugs. Your general practitioner may refer you to a psychiatrist or a psychologist for assessment and possibly for treatment.

You might be in a different position from most other people, if you are already linked in with a psychiatric service, with an educational service or with a charity that you attend regularly for care in relation to your autism spectrum disorder. These services usually assign a key-worker or a contact person within a multi-disciplinary team to each client. In this case, if you have a key-worker or counsellor who you trust, then you might want to discuss any difficult health-related issues you have with that trusted person first. Your counsellor or key-worker is not necessarily going to be able to help with the issue, but may well have good knowledge about the issue and about who would be best to consult about it.

7.1.2 Consultants

Consultants are people who have spent additional time learning a medical speciality and training in that speciality in a clinical setting, like a hospital, under guidance of qualified specialists. There are specialists in almost everything, such as cancer diagnosis, gastro-enterology, neurology or psychiatry. In most cases you would access specialist diagnosis or treatment through your general practitioner — they write a letter of referral, and you then receive an appointment with the consultant. You might be given a choice between a public appointment through an HSE-employed consultant or a private consultant. A private appointment will usually be sooner. You will have to pay for a private consultation but, if you have private health insurance, then it will probably cover some or all of the fees. Sometimes the consultant will be the same person (occasionally in the same hospital), because consultants often see both public and private patients, but preserve enough of their time to provide earlier appointments for patients willing to pay.

If you are an adult and not yet diagnosed, then you will have to pay for assessment by a private consultant psychiatrist. If you have private health insurance, then it may cover some or all of the fees for private assessment. Whether you have insurance or not, you can claim income tax relief for medical expenses that have not been reimbursed by any other source.

In most cases you will need to attend consultant appointments in their own hospital or private consulting rooms. They may arrange separate appointments for diagnostic tests, especially time-consuming tests like MRI or endoscopy, and might not see you on the day of the test — you may have to wait for the results to be processed and sent back to your general practitioner. Sometimes a test will exclude any illness (in which case your general practitioner will tell you the results) and sometimes they will indicate the need for further tests or a consultation with the specialist.

If you need to see a consultant or have tests, then you can minimise the stress and disruption by making yourself familiar with what to expect (they sometimes send a description of the procedure to your general practitioner, or you may find a leaflet on most common procedures in the doctor's surgery) and planning your time and journey in advance. Some procedures will make it impossible to drive (including some eye-tests involving dilation of the pupil of the eye, which affects vision for several hours) and some will require that somebody accompanies you on your journey home (such as endoscopy, which uses drugs that affect balance and memory). Planning your journey and writing down all the times, the bus or train details and phone numbers of people you might need to contact will provide reassurance, even if you do not need to refer to any of it. In many cases, the simplest solution is to use a local minicab company that you trust to collect you from the hospital — you will need to have their phone number with you and might prefer to ask a receptionist or a medic to call on your behalf to explain the details to them, especially if you feel or sound light-headed or woozy.

7.1.3 The Accident and Emergency department

The Accident and Emergency department in a hospital exists to deal with serious medical issues that require urgent medical care. Sometimes these may be relatively minor things that need diagnostic tests or treatment that is only available in a hospital (injuries that might be a sprain or a broken bone, or diarrhoea with dehydration). Other times it will be obvious when emergency treatment is needed — for example serious workplace injuries or injuries in car accidents. The Accident and Emergency departments of most hospitals are heavily used and under-resourced, so there is a system of triage involving inspection of the injury or a description of symptoms soon after arrival. The most urgent cases are dealt with soonest and less urgent cases wait longer — it is common to wait several hours or even overnight in an Accident and Emergency department, during which time you may be asked to undergo several tests (such as X-ray or blood tests) and to wait while the results are processed. Although Accident and Emergency is a part of the public Health Service Executive, there is a fee (currently €100) for each 'episode' of attendance — in some cases, you might be sent home and asked to return after a test has been processed or a consultant is available, but this will count as one episode of treatment and one fee. There is a general view that Accident and Emergency treatment is misused by patients who avoid paying their general practitioner for consultations and use the hospital instead when they feel very ill, and the fee is partly to discourage misuse.

The Accident and Emergency department is also the first place to call for serious, urgent emotional or psychiatric issues — for instance strong feelings that involve thoughts of suicide or harming another person, or episodes of violent rage that are frightening. It is also the place to go to when if you have deliberately injured yourself (for instance by cutting), or taken overdose of drugs — whether deliberate or accidental. Accident and Emergency departments can treat the immediate injury or poisoning and refer to an on-call psychiatrist for an assessment of any mood disorder. This applies even if you have **not** injured yourself in any way — if you feel the need to injure yourself, or have thoughts about killing yourself, then the Accident and Emergency department is open all day and all night.

7.2 VHI and private health insurance

Ireland has a unique mix of a public health system, private health care, private health insurance and a semi-state health insurer. The semi-state health insurer, VHI (the Voluntary Health Insurance Board), currently operates under principles that require it to provide health insurance to all customers on equal terms — irrespective of age, health, previous illness or insurance history. Health insurance is available on equal terms to any person who can pay the premium. This means, for instance, that people who would be considered a bad insurance risk because they are old or diagnosed with a lifelong medical condition can also buy health insurance at the same premium. The largest private health insurer, Aviva, is obliged to commercially compete with the VHI for customers, keeping health insurance premiums lower in Ireland than in many other countries. The future of the VHI is not certain, and has been challenged by private health insurers and the European Union, who would like insurers to compete on an equal commercial basis. For the present, most health insurance in Ireland is broadly similar and nobody can be refused health insurance or charged higher premiums because of previous illness.

Health insurance is banded from "One" or "Plan A" that provides basic cover, up to "HealthPlus Platinum" or "Plan E" that also covers your personal choice of most private consultants operating in Ireland as well as cover for a wider range of issues. The majority of people use the first or second levels ("One+" or "Plan B") of insurance. Health insurance is sold as a family product, covering all the people in one household, and including financial dependents such as children who are still in full-time education, such as third-level students. Many employers provide health insurance cover to their employees, or have an option to buy private health insurance from salary — an employer's policy will be cheaper than personal insurance, and may provide additional benefits. Most insurers also offer separate dental and travel health insurance — although it is worth remembering that Irish residents are covered for treatment in most countries of the European Union, and you can request a European Health Insurance Card from the HSE to use when accessing treatments such as Accident and Emergency or doctors while on holiday or short-term employment in Europe.

7.2.1 Services covered by insurance

You must read all the terms of any insurance policy you consider buying or consider using. You must check that your policy covers you for the types of treatment that you currently use, or that you have good reason to imagine that you might need in the future. You may need to do some financial accounting of how much you are spending on health care to decide which level of policy will save you money, or provide the greatest security against potential health costs.

Higher levels of policy include cover for occupational therapy, physiotherapy and other kinds of non-hospital medical treatment that are not covered by the basic level policy. You do not have a free choice of therapist because they must have appropriate qualifications and registration. In some cases they must also appear on a list of practitioners approved by the insurer.

Complementary and alternative therapies are generally not covered by insurance, although there has been a move towards providing cover for therapies that patients claim are effective — even when scientific research does not show a consistent positive effect. Happy patients get better faster and at lower cost and choice makes patients happy. Insurers will not cover patients for therapies that are harmful.

7.3 Privacy and intimate topics

Going to a doctor or other medical professional will often require you to reveal intimate details about your life or your symptoms, or allow yourself to be examined in areas that you normally keep private. Sometimes these will make you feel uncomfortable or embarrassed, and some intimate physical examinations may raise intense discomfort or upset. Some people will avoid talking about their medical problems, especially if they think that the doctor might want to look at or touch parts of their body that are normally private. These reactions are entirely normal, but it is very important that you do discuss your medical issues and have your symptoms examined, both to avoid physical and emotional distress of being unwell and to ensure that your symptoms do not become worse.

Remember that doctors have seen absolutely everything before and there is very little that will surprise, shock or offend a doctor — but obviously you should not intentionally try to do so. Sexually-transmitted infections are very widespread, despite the availability of effective treatments, because people who have symptoms related to urination and their genitals are too embarrassed to talk to their doctors about — or to visit a sexual health clinic away from home. The medical profession would much prefer to see and treat these conditions, which cause distress that far exceeds the embarrassment of talking about or allowing the doctor to see private parts.

Other problems that people often avoid talking to a doctor about are bowel function, bleeding when passing stools, body odour, discharge and itching or rashes. Most of these are caused by inconsequential conditions that can be treated very easily with prescription drugs, but can also be signs of problems that might be more serious. There are many over-the-counter drugs and ointments that help reduce symptoms like pain, itching or abnormal bleeding — but these symptoms should always be assessed to check that you are not masking a treatable problem.

Many people also avoid talking about their emotions and state of mind, especially when they feel depressed or when they think that the feelings are signs of 'madness'. You might be surprised that many, many people worry about signs of madness and are worried about telling anyone. Depression and worry can become a self-promoting cycle that gets worse and worse, with increasing avoidance of other people or talking about the problem. If you need to talk about problems that are worrying or frightening and really can not talk to your doctor, you could instead talk to a student counsellor if you are in school or college, to the Samaritans (anonymously if you prefer) or to a mental health helpline run by Aware, Grow or Shine. There are more specific helplines like the Rape Crisis Centre or Childline if you need to talk to someone about sexual or physical abuse issues that are worrying you. These types of worries can sometimes become serious many years after the events, and Childline also talks to adults who have worries about neglect and abuse in their childhood ('historical abuse').

7.3.1 Intimate conversations

If you do need to discuss an intimate issue with a doctor, then it can help to write down the issues that you need to talk about. Whether these are emotional issues, relationship problems or physical symptoms, it will help a great deal to have a set of words that describe your issues. Do not worry about using the correct medical terms, just use the ones that you are comfortable saying. These might be the correct Latin terms, the words you use with your parents (it does not matter if they sound childish) or the slang you use with your friends. There are some slang words that are very offensive, so use them if it is the only word you know, but use words which are less offensive if you can. Use a dictionary or an internet search if you do not know the words you need.

A short list of items can be helpful too. If you find it too hard to say the things that you need to say, then you can hand the list to the doctor to read and to prompt you for further information if it is necessary. You should not expect your doctor to want to read lengthy descriptions, pages full of detail or pages of possible diagnoses that you have downloaded from the internet — a short list of words on a sticky note, or one side of a sheet of paper should be sufficient.

Remember that doctors have seen and heard almost everything before, and the problem you have is getting the conversation started about your own specific issues. If you are unable to raise the issues yourself, then talk them over with a relative or friend who you are comfortable with and ask that person to come with you into the consultation to talk for you.

Doctors might need to ask questions about your behaviour, your activities and your diet that you find personal and intrusive. These questions are almost always in your own best interests, so try to answer them as accurately and honestly as you can.

7.3.2 Intimate procedures

Doctors need to look at symptoms to see what they are and how severe they are — 'a swelling' can mean different things to different people, and needs to be assessed properly. This is usually fine if the doctor only needs to look at a hand or in your ear, but can be difficult if there is significant physical contact or if you need to undress.

A significant issue for some people with autism spectrum disorder is that touch can be distressing, and the sensory issues of bright light, the smell of disinfectant and having an object put inside your mouth, or elsewhere, can lead to overload. Sometimes this can cause you to become extremely distressed or emotional. If you know that this happens with you, then talk to the doctor about it before the examination to give warning of what to expect and to explain why it is happening. Asking for a tissue can be a simple way of indicating that you are upset and about to cry, without having to explain anything — doctor's surgeries always have tissues.

If you are frightened of being touched inappropriately, or unsure about what is or is not appropriate, then you can ask someone to come into the consultation with you. No reasonable doctor will refuse the request.

Some men have a fear that they will get an erection during a medical examination of their penis, testes or rectum. Like everything else, the doctor has seen it all before.

7.3.3 If you are not comfortable with your particular doctor

If you are not comfortable with your particular doctor, or do not feel able to talk about intimate issues or to be touched or examined by your particular doctor, then you should consider changing to another doctor. It will really help you to examine why you feel uncomfortable so that you can choose an appropriate doctor to change to. One common reason is that you would feel more comfortable with a doctor of the same sex or the opposite sex as yourself, or a doctor close to or far from your own age. There may be some specific issues about the doctor's attitudes or behaviour that you do not like, or some non-specific issues that you can not specific but feel uncomfortable about. There may be issues specific to yourself, such as your sexual orientation or identity that would make you choose a doctor that you can talk to about those issues. Whatever the reason, being able to identify what you need in a doctor is key to finding the right doctor for you, and to avoid changing doctor's repeatedly in the hope of finding the right doctor. If you are able to discuss your reasons for wanting to change with your current doctor, then it is very likely that your current doctor can suggest suitable choices to you.

7.4 Some common medical issues

There are several common problems that bring people to their doctors, and some of these can cause repeated visits. Exercise and a healthy diet are something that most people do not manage as well as they could. Adequate exercise and a healthy diet improve physical and mental health in very many ways, and they have a lifelong impact. Some common problems that can result in repeated visits to the doctor and a great deal of distress include irritable bowel syndrome (IBS), being overweight, sexually-transmitted infections, poor sleep, sexual dysfunction and pain that does not go away. Although none of these is caused by autism spectrum disorder, there can be a strong interaction between emotional and sensory issues that mean the quality of life is affected more for someone with autism.

Some of these common medical problems are of particular

interest for people who are not fully in touch with emotions. The body and mind interact so that emotional states create matching physical states, and vice versa. If you are emotionally upset (even if you do not recognize the emotional upset), then you may feel physically unwell. If you are physically unwell, then you may become depressed. These psychosomatic (mind-body) interactions are very real, and they are not signs of hypochondria or 'imaginary' illnesses — a psychosomatic illness is as real as any other, and just as uncomfortable or painful. A physical illness may sometimes be nature's way of telling you that you are not attending to emotional stresses.

7.4.1 Exercise, diet and well-being

Exercise and a healthy diet affect mental health as well as physical health. Governments regularly publish guidelines on recommended levels of moderate and vigorous physical activity. Adults are recommended to take at least 150 minutes (30 minutes on 5 different days) of moderate activity per week. Moderate activities include brisk walking, gardening, swimming, cycling, and dancing. Vigorous activity provides the same benefit in half the time, so adults should have at least 75 minutes (15 minutes on 5 different days) of vigorous activity. Vigorous activities are things that raise your heart rate and breathing, and they include Jogging, running, team sports, aerobics, circuit training, rowing, paced swimming, brisk dancing, skipping and hill-walking or climbing. Physical activity can be a part of work and routine — such as taking the stairs instead of the lift, or walking to a more distant shop.

Diet should be balanced, moderate and varied. We discuss some specific issues in Chapter 4 because diet can be a problem for some people with autism, because the need for routine and the sensory issues that some people with autism have can make it difficult to obtain a healthy balance. There is no mystery in healthy diet — do not eat nutritionally poor foods to excess and do eat plenty of fresh fruit and vegetables. Nutritionally poor foods include most snack foods, convenience foods, sweets and anything that is high in fat, high in sugar or high in salt and flavourings.

7.4.2 Irritable bowel syndrome

Irritable bowel syndrome is a **functional disorder** of the digestive tract, which means that it is a syndrome diagnosed by a collection of symptoms, but it has no organic cause. Between 10% and 15% of the population may have irritable bowel syndrome. The functional symptoms include diarrhoea, constipation, abdominal pain, weight loss, blood in the faeces (hematochezia), infection and various signs of upper and lower gastrointestinal inflammation. Diarrhoea and constipation may alternate, or even be present in the same bowel movement. Tests and investigations will rule out identifiable disease, food intolerance or metabolic disorders, leaving the diagnosis of irritable bowel syndrome. There is no cure for irritable bowel syndrome, but some therapies can help to manage the difficulties that it causes.

Note that any blood in the faeces should be assessed to determine its cause — whether hematochezia (bright, fresh blood due to irritable bowel syndrome), bleeding from piles or darker blood from bleeding in the small intestine or stomach.

There is no scientific evidence that gastrointestinal problems are more common in people with autism, but there are good reasons to accept that emotional upset and sensory difficulties interact with the emotional and physical distress caused by irritable bowel syndrome. People with autism may be affected to a greater degree by physical pain and emotional stress certainly contributes to the frequency of gastrointestinal upsets, so the interaction may work in both directions. Managing irritable bowel syndrome may have a greater impact on quality of life for someone who also has autism.

Diet is the most effective therapy for irritable bowel syndrome, particularly the management of dietary and supplementary fibres. Soluble fibre (including supplements) can reduce symptoms, whilst insoluble fibre (such as bran) is ineffective and may even aggravate the symptoms. Some foods and beverages — tea, coffee, smoking, alcohol, chocolate and some spices — are known irritants that should be consumed in moderation or avoided.

Drugs that may help include laxatives (such as lactulose, or polyethylene glycol or PEG) for constipation, anti-diarrhoeals, antispasmodics and domperidone for bloating and abdominal pain, as well as tricyclic antidepressants, serotonin agonists and selective serotonin re-uptake inhibitors (SSRIs). Over-use of over-the-counter drugs and self-medication with supplements or other remedies can mask symptoms of inflammation and infections resulting from irritable bowel syndrome.

7.4.3 Diet and weight-loss

Most people in Ireland are overweight. In a recent survey, — 61% were overweight and 24% were obese. Being overweight is a consequence of eating too much and exercising too little, but is far more than a dietary issue because it involves mental well-being, self-esteem and issues about control and autonomy. People eat for comfort and eat in combination with their lifestyle and circumstances. Food choices can be limited by unemployment, overwork, leisure choices and your circle of friends.

Losing weight requires that you reduce your calorie intake from your diet below the amount expended by your physical activity and (the most difficult part) keeping the intake that low for months, for years or a lifetime. Losing weight and maintaining healthy weight means making a permanent lifestyle change to your diet, your activity or to both. There are no quick fixes to weight loss and maintenance — although there is no end to the diets, fads, food supplements and books about dieting and slimming. Almost any diet will help a healthy person to lose weight, but the one ingredient that a successful weight management regime requires is long-term commitment.

A healthy weight is often measured by body mass index (BMI), defined as your weight (in kilograms) divided by the square of your height (in meters) — for instance a man who weighs 90 kilograms and is 1.8 meters tall has a body mass index of 27.8 (90 divided by 3.24). A body mass index of 25 or more is considered to be overweight and 30 or more is considered obese, so this man would be overweight, but he would not be obese. There are several different methods of estimating adiposity (being overweight), which academics have endless arguments over. But even if one version puts you over or under the magic threshold, a measurement of 24.9 or 25.1 means you are either at the heavy end of the normal range or slightly overweight, which both mean that you should take care of your exercise and food intake. Some alternative measures of being overweight include a waist size of more than 94cm (37 inches) for men and more than 80cm (31.5 inches) for women, or a waist-to-hip ratio of more than 1.0 for men and more than 0.8 for women. Any one of these methods is adequate for monitoring your own health over time.

7.4.4 Sexually-transmitted infections

Sexually-transmitted infections include genital warts, herpes, gonorrhoea, syphilis, hepatitis and HIV. HPV, which causes some cervical cancers, is also sexually-transmitted. All of these infections can be passed through sexual contact, particularly when bodily fluids are exchanged. They can all cause serious health effects, including discomfort, pain, infertility, neurological damage and, if left untreated, can be fatal. Sexual transmission of infection can be greatly reduced by using a barrier method of contraception (condom) and both partners should take responsibility for their personal health.

You can discuss any problems that you think might be related to sexual health with your own doctor, or with several other professionals. Problems include an unusual discharge from your penis or vagina (even if it does not have a bad odour), pain when urinating, sores or blisters on your genitals, anus or nearby, unusual pain during sexual intercourse and blood in your urine. If you do not want to talk about these symptoms or your sexual behaviour with your own doctor, it is still vital that you talk to someone. Sexual health clinics are listed as STI or GUM (genito-urinary medicine) clinics, Well-woman clinics or Well-man clinics. All third level institutes and the Irish Family Planning Association also run sexual health clinics.

7.4.5 Insomnia and sleep hygiene

Insomnia is the persistent lack of good quality sleep, leading to day-time tiredness and frequent, restless napping or drowsiness. Some insomnia is the result of physical causes, such as snoring, night-time noise, a poor sleep environment or ill-health causing pain or discomfort. Some insomnia is the result of emotional disturbances such as anxiety and depression. Poor sleep has a big impact on quality of life, daytime alertness and learning or working abilities. Do not interfere with your sleep patterns if you have no problems with your sleep — there is no reason to fix something that is not broken.

Sleep hygiene is a term that refers to the methodical construction of a routine and an environment that helps you to get good quality sleep. It is necessary to structure both the routine of resting and the environment in which you rest to solve problems with your sleep.

Constructing a good sleep environment involves creating a place where you rest and sleep, with as little distraction by activities that raise your alertness. A bedroom and a bed should be used for sleep (and for sex), but for no other activity — do not watch television, use your laptop computer, play video games, have late-night discussions or make telephone calls from your bed. These all cause physical and emotional arousal, and you need to break the association between alertness and the place that you sleep.

Create routine around your sleep, which includes going to bed at the same time every day. It does not matter when this time is, which will vary greatly from one person to another. If you are consistently tired or have difficulty waking in the morning, then it should probably be earlier than you currently go to bed. If you are not tired, then do not go to bed. If you go to bed and feel restless, then get out of bed and do something relaxing and calming, such as reading a novel or listening to calm music, until you do feel tired — but remember that going to bed late does not excuse you from getting up on time the next day. Routine includes getting up at the same time every day, especially when you do not feel like it, and that time must be early enough to provide you with the potential for a productive day and the potential to interact with the people you should be interacting with — especially people who you share a home with, but also colleagues or potential colleagues. Not being awake and alert when somebody calls will immediately remove opportunity from your life. Try not to catnap, to doze during the daytime or to sleep in the afternoon. All of these take away from the routine of sleeping at sleeping time and being alert during waking time.

Some foods interfere with sleep. Coffee, tea and chocolate contain stimulants that will keep you awake. Coffee and tea are also diuretic, which means that make you need to urinate more or sooner. These beverages and alcohol are irritants that will make you want to empty your bladder even when it is not full, especially if you have cystitis or any kind of urinary tract infection. Some people claim that certain foods — cheese is often blamed — cause restlessness and bad dreams. This is probably not strictly true, but eating or drinking close to bedtime will cause abdominal discomfort during the night. You should eat your evening meal with a few hours to digest before bed, and not drink any fluids within an hour or two of bedtime. Alcohol in particular causes disturbed and poor quality sleep because it makes you feel sleepy, but interferes with breathing and comfort.

Placing your hands inside the bedclothes has an effect on circulation that helps the whole body to relax and sleep. Our circulatory system responds to cold as a potential threat and increases blood-flow to the vital organs, including the brain, and raises vigilance. Being comfortably warm, with adequate ventilation in the room, is most conducive to good sleep. It is better to have plenty of warm bedclothes in a cool room than to have a stuffy or over-warm environment — even in sleep, you will be able to move and expose more or less of your body to control your body temperature.

7.4.6 Sexual dysfunction

Sexual health has been defined as having the sex that you want — including none — in a safe way, without risk of harming yourself or others physically or emotionally. Within this definition of sexual health, there is an immense range of behaviours from asexual to a varied sex life that are all 'normal'. When emotional or physical ill-health interferes with the ability to have the sex that you want to have, then this may lead to sexual dysfunction. The most widely-recognized sexual dysfunction is erectile dysfunction (also called impotence), when a man is unable to get an erection or to sustain an erection during sexual activity. Sexual dysfunction also includes a lack of arousal and anorgasmia (difficulty reaching orgasm or ejaculation). Sometimes sexual dysfunction can have a physical cause, sometimes it is emotional or psychological, and sometimes a combination of the two.

There are drugs such as Viagra that can help a man to have and maintain an erection when the cause is primarily a physical one. These drugs are prescription drugs available by consultation with your doctor or a sexual health or Well-man clinic. There are very many unlicensed products claiming to have similar effects, most of which have not been adequately tested or are simply ineffective. Some unlicensed products are harmful or contain active ingredients of other drugs not intended for sexual dysfunction. There are experimental drugs to increase arousal and libido in women (including prostaglandin and testosterone), but none has yet not been approved for general use.

Emotional and psychological reasons for lack of sexual arousal and reduced libido include situational anorgasmia or situational erectile dysfunction — arousal and orgasm are fine in one situation (e.g. when masturbating), but can not be achieved in another (e.g. with your partner). Sometimes this can be very literally situational, such as not being able to achieve orgasm in your childhood home, even as an adult. Sometimes it is the combination of conscious and unconscious fears and anxieties that accompany sexual activity only in combination with your partner. Talking therapies as an individual or as a couple can effectively uncover those issues and lead to a more satisfying sexual experience. Remember that you do not **have to perform** sexually, and certainly not to somebody else's schedule and standards — performance anxiety is a cold shower for your libido.

Women who experience anorgasmia with a partner have found devices like the Hitachi Magic Wand have helped them to achieve satisfying orgasm, alone or with their partner. These are vibrating massagers that are not designed for insertion into the vagina, so stimulation is directed towards the vulva and the clitoris, rather than attempting to stimulate by penetration. Most pornographic and other images of female sexual response revolve around penetration, which many men (and even women) assume is required for satisfying sex. Adopting more gentle techniques, with a slower introduction, helps many women to find sex more stimulating and more satisfying.

7.4.7 Pain

Some people suffer from chronic pain and from episodes of acute pain that can be extremely disruptive and distressing. These include cluster headaches, migraine, as well as chronic pain that does not respond to treatment (intractable pain). Self-medication with over-the-counter drugs — especially those drugs containing codeine — can both mask the underlying illness and lead to additional problems caused by inappropriate drug use.

There are treatments for cluster headaches and for migraine, but they do not work for everyone. Migraine can lead to nausea, light-sensitivity, 'aura' (a halo or geometric images in your field of view) and over-reaction to noise or touch. Catching the migraine early is one of the most useful management techniques, because lying down in a quiet and darkened room may be enough to avoid a full-blown migraine without any drugs, or only using aspirin or paracetamol. No over-the-counter remedy is effective once a migraine has started, but there are some powerful prescription-only treatments that some individuals find very effective.

Chronic pain — such as trigeminal neuralgia or peripheral neuropathic pain — can be caused by previous illness (chickenpox can damage nerves, as can some vibrating machine tools or repeated exposure to chemicals like cement), or have no identifiable cause. Some people may respond to particular drugs, particular combinations of drugs, or drugs in combination with exercise and relaxation. A number of anti-depressant drugs (some tricyclics and serotonin-norepinephrine re-uptake inhibitors or SNRIs) and some anti-epileptics have side-effects that reduce nervous system pain — they are prescribed specifically for this pain-management side-effect, not because the doctor believes you are depressed or epileptic. Surveys have found that between 10% and 30% of the population suffer from some form of chronic pain, but despite this prevalence, modern medicine is very ineffective at managing pain. Successful management of long-term pain will involve prescription drugs when these do help, in combination with lifestyle changes that minimize exposure to stressors that trigger episodes of pain and therapies that promote relaxation and emotional well-being. Pain is far more bearable and far more manageable when you are happy than when you are tense or when you are sad.

Sometimes pain can have distinct, repeating patterns or associations with particular activities — if you think to look for them. One common example is the weekend migraine, where you are fine during the week and then have severe migraines in what should be your own leisure and relaxation time, perhaps every Saturday morning. These can indicate that work is extremely pressured or stressful. If you have difficulty in understanding and describing your own feelings (alexithymia), then it may be the first indication that you notice of problems like workplace bullying or unreasonable work demands. It may simply be your body's way of telling your brain that you are unhappy.

7.5 Hypochondria

Hypochondria is technically an **excessive** anxiety or preoccupation with ill-health or symptoms, but is also used colloquially to refer to having a low threshold for seeking medical care, even for trivial problems. People who have a lifelong diagnosed condition, such as an autism spectrum disorder, will naturally tend to see their doctor and to have more medical tests, so they may feel that they are excessively seeking medical attention when it is actually an essential component of their lives.

People who have a lifelong diagnosed condition are also likely to have higher levels of depression and anxiety, which can make every symptom seem more significant and more serious than it really is. This is closer to a real hypochondria, but is also a natural consequence of having a condition that is perceived as being a medical disorder.

If you are feel that you are a hypochondriac and seek excessive medical attention, then discuss it with your doctor or someone else that you trust. It is likely that your doctor will tell you to continue seeking advice, and that it is better to be safe than sorry.

8 Managing the barriers to doing (*Diarmuid Heffernan*)

The purpose of this chapter is to assist you in dealing with the numerous points of contact with bureaucracy and the people in various public services that you will come into contact with in your life. We will also look at why you may find certain actions necessary in your life difficult to do and how you may address and cope with this, including sources of support and people who can help you. The examples we will focus on here are issues such as Social Welfare, Tax and managing money but also includes healthcare, job applications, submitting coursework and the fear, procrastination or perfectionism you may experience which can impinge on your ability to cope with these necessities.

The primary question we asked ourselves in beginning to write this chapter is why might someone with an ASD need assistance with issues of bureaucracy or dealing with public services/servants. The main issue is that ASDs are associated with some social and cognitive differences (as set out in chapter one) that make social, civic and bureaucratic functions difficult, and these differences are lifelong — therefore many people with ASDs need support in addressing these issues.

8.1 Procrastination

One of the manifestations of the difficulties people with ASD face, in our experience, is a tendency to procrastinate around bureaucratic issues. For example, replying to a letter from the Revenue (or college, banks, employers etc). Many people feel intimidated by the thoughts of interacting with these institutions and the people that represent them and thus become anxious at the thoughts of replying or responding to them and put it off. The difficulty with this is that these institutions will expect or need a response (even if they are asking a relatively innocuous question) and will generally continue to contact you until they get a reply. It is also fair to say that many people find bureaucratic language intimidating and organisations often follow procedures no matter what!

We would suggest that there are ways of dealing with this type of bureaucracy which may allow you to control your own levels of anxiety around it and feel secure in responding. The first thing we would suggest is purchasing folders or a filing cabinet (or both), or having a space in an existing cupboard etc where you can file correspondence from banks, Revenue, Office of Social Protection and also bills, rent receipts etc. It is advisable to separate the various correspondence out, and file in different folders devoted only to each category. This may also be done on your computer by creating a folder or folders devoted to such correspondence. Having categorised and separated correspondence/bills etc out it is then very important that you respond and deal with each (rather than just filing them away without action — out of sight out of mind!). We suggest that the best way to do this is through the creation of a routine. This routine should focus on dealing with letters or correspondence as you receive them. If necessary use your calendar (online or paper) to remind yourself of the things you need to respond to. The creation of this routine takes effort and toil but ultimately it will make things much easier on yourself. Though it may feel tempting and easier to put off dealing with bureaucracy, we feel that it in fact creates more anxiety for you and the anxiety of actually responding to correspondence may often become the issue rather than what may be contained in the correspondence you need to reply to.

8.2 Intimidation

The second reason we feel people might find it difficult to deal with bureaucracy is feeling intimidated. For example, Revenue, the Department of Social Protection and other public services/institutions may contact you directly by phone with queries. For many people this can be intimidating or overwhelming, particularly if it is unexpected. There may be a variety of reasons why people may find the thoughts of this type of interaction so difficult. For instance it may be because it is a fear of the unknown, what this person may say that you are not prepared for (the unexpected). It may be because of a lack of social imagination and an inability to see what the person might say, how they might say it, or why. For many people with ASDs it's because these types of interaction contain too many uncontrollable variables and therefore become risky (a fear of saying the wrong thing and appearing foolish or incompetent is often an issue for people with or without an ASD). For others it's the intimidation of perceived authority. In reality, most people with an ASD find these interactions difficult because of some if not all of the above reasons, as well as other social-cultural factors which may influence how we view Government and authority (for example our colonial past and its links to distrust/dislike of authority). There are ways of combating the fears and anxieties regarding these types of interactions.

Our advice is that you do not have to answer questions on the phone if you are feeling too anxious or overwhelmed. You can politely ask the person who has contacted you for a contact number where you can ring them back or if they could call you the following day. This is not a way of procrastinating but rather a way of preparing yourself for dealing with the person and their queries etc. It may be helpful for you to write down what you need to say to the person or indeed the reply to their query (depending on who you are talking to this may also include writing a list of questions for the person you are dealing with, it may also be advisable to have account numbers etc written down so that you don't have to go looking for the details). If you feel able to do so you can explain that you find the phone call difficult because you are anxious (we certainly would not advise this in general phone correspondence as it is not advisable to divulge personal information if it is not appropriate).

A further way of preparing yourself for dealing with bureaucracy or public services is to do online research into your rights and entitlements and the purpose of various agencies. For example the Citizens Information website (www.citizensinformation.ie/) or the Revenue website (www.revenue.ie/) are both very useful sites. It is also worth noting that you can make appointments with various public servants, for example, tax inspectors, if you prefer to deal with them directly rather than via phone or e mail.

If you have trusted friends/partners/family members or advocates then it may be wise to consult with them if you have difficulties as set out above, these trusted people can contact organisations on your behalf. It is important at this juncture to say that we as authors of this book feel that there is a distinct gap in services in Ireland who advocate for or support adults with ASDs. This is not to stigmatise or assume disability in people on the Autism spectrum, on the contrary we acknowledge and celebrate difference and indeed the positive and vital contribution of people with ASDs to society. It is merely a recognition of the benefits people with ASDs may get from the support and advocacy of services which may help with issues such as we are describing in this chapter and throughout the book.

8.3 Sensory issues in bureaucratic spaces

The third reason we feel people with ASDs might find it difficult in dealing with bureaucracy is the sensory and interactive issues associated with certain spaces. For example, the reality of most Social Welfare offices in Ireland at this moment is that they are crowded and potentially difficult spaces to be in. It is important to try not to let this dissuade you from going, but it is also important to know what you may be facing. Generally the interior of Social Welfare offices are not architecturally or aesthetically pleasing, rather they are designed to be functional. The offices may also contain many sensory components that you may find difficult to contend with. One such component is crowds of people, another is the commensurate noise created by crowds, there may also be other smells such as body odors, strong perfume/aftershave, certain materials/clothing etc or issues of proximity to others in a queue, for example, that you find difficult. Some people have an object that they use to comfort themselves with when they are feeling anxious, for example some people carry beads in their pocket which they can hold without others knowing they are doing it. It is fair to say that this has its limits. If someone uses a large incongruous object publicly this may attract unwanted attention (we are not saying not to do it, rather we feel you should be aware that the consequence of doing it will most likely be increased attention and potentially negative attention from those around you). Another coping strategy may be to have some headphones on with calming music, or some people use a repeated mantra for themselves such as "I will be calm", etc until it is your turn to talk with staff. It is our experience that in most instances staff in Social Welfare offices are reasonable and approachable, therefore try not to let the less than salubrious surroundings put you off!

8.4 Planning and preparation

If you do need to deal directly (face to face) with a public service, there are a number of strategies you can use that may make this a less stressful situation. For example, it may be worthwhile writing down any questions you may have regarding payments or entitlements or any other queries you may have, plus all your facts — Date of Birth, phone number, address, account numbers — which all may be helpful if you find yourself clamming up or losing your speech due to anxiety. In this instance you may also choose to tell the person you are dealing with that you are anxious if you feel able to do so. If you do not have a trusted advocate in these situations it is very important to be able to advocate for yourself and this is why we encourage you to try to overcome anxieties around dealing, either directly or indirectly, with public services or bureaucracy.

The act of writing down questions or important points is generally a very useful exercise and a potentially good habit to get into.

Apart from the reasons set out above, another good reason to write down things you need to ask/do etc is because many of us have a poor working memory (including and especially both authors of this book!). Having a poor working memory means forgetting potentially important things during the course of a day or week and can lead to forgetting about doctor's appointments, paying bills or other important times/dates. We have discussed in various chapters the benefits of having a calendar either online or on your wall or both. It may also be very useful to put reminders on your phone as well as purchasing a diary with important dates etc written in. It is good practice to write reminders in as they occur or as they occur to you i.e. when you remember them! By writing these down as they occur you bypass the difficulties of a poor working memory and rely on your reminders to guide you. It is advisable you write reminders down as they occur because you cannot be certain you will remember to write them down later! (as has often happened to this author). So write reminders as they occur to you and it is acceptable in almost any social situation to ask the person you are talking with if they mind you writing a note. Most people will understand the necessity for making reminders.

8.5 Anxiety in public spaces

The final reason we feel that many people with an ASD may put off dealing with bureaucracy is to do with perceptions they may have of the people in the office etc who are also waiting to be seen, or the people they may pass/encounter on their way to the Dole office etc (This anxiety associated with other people in public spaces can often prevent people with ASDs from leaving their homes for almost any reason other than essentials such as shopping and can cause the person to become isolated. This is often why people with ASDs are perceived to prefer their own company. It is often not a preference but a stark choice between extreme anxiety and isolation). One of these perceptions revolves around the concept of ideas of reference. This means in essence that the person with an ASD may feel that those around them are talking about them. An example of this may be that you are walking down a busy street and are feeling stressed, anxious or possibly a little overwhelmed by the sensory stimuli you are facing. As you become more anxious you may start to feel that people are focusing in on you, either by staring at you or by saying things to each other about you. This may even manifest in hearing people say your name as they walk by. This is both a side effect of anxiety (and possibly bad experiences in the past such as bullying or ostracisation) and also a further cause of anxiety. In reality most people on the streets of bigger cities in particular do not pay much heed to others. This may not alleviate your feeling that they are, however.

One way of dealing with this issue is by acknowledging that you are feeling stressed and accepting the likelihood that strangers on the street are not particularly focused in on you and are not saying your name, and the sense you have that they are is based on your own anxiety (though if you are very anxious and your body language is clearly showing this then it may attract people's attention in public). There are other ways of counteracting these feelings. One is to wear headphones with soothing music or mantras playing. Another is to avoid streets or areas of streets which are particularly busy or noisy or where people are more likely to congregate. A further way of combating these feelings is by talking to a trusted person in your life about them. We would advise caution in this regard as it may appear to others that what you are describing is 'strange' or even 'psychotic' thinking. It is very important therefore to talk to someone that you know will listen without judgement. If you are attending counselling, or contemplating attending counselling, it may be worthwhile seeking a counsellor with experience of working with people with ASDs. In presenting these difficulties to others it may be best to frame it in the context of anxiety that is context-specific, in other words that certain situations make you more anxious — for instance being in crowded streets.

If there are ways of soothing or comforting yourself during these situations then there may be ways of doing so without drawing undue attention on yourself. For example having a comforting item to touch or hold in your pocket. Many people with ASDs derive comfort by talking to themselves. If spoken out loud this may attract unwanted attention so a creative way of avoiding unwanted attention is by having a bluetooth earpiece in your ear which makes it appear as if you are having a telephone conversation with someone.

A second way in which many people with ASDs may perceive others is through perceived intent. This means you may have a sense that others mean harm or have malice towards you. This usually manifests in public spaces, particularly where there are crowds of people and it can be a distressing experience. It may also be linked with anxiety and stress or past experiences. It can be a distressing experience but can also potentially be a limiting one as it may prevent you from going places or doing things where this feeling may occur. An example of how it may occur is when passing a group of people congregated in a particular area, you may get a sense of malice or intent of harm towards you from the group.

It is important you try and combat this by reassuring yourself that incidents of violence in public spaces are quite rare, are usually between people who already know each other and are fuelled by alcohol or other drugs. These incidents are also far more likely to occur in particular areas and at particular times, therefore for the most part the vast majority of people will never experience unprovoked attacks from strangers. There are some common sense ways of avoiding potential flashpoints such as staying in well lit busy streets at night, ignoring drunken ranting which may be aimed indiscriminately at whoever happens to be nearest at the time, particularly late at night, and walking around rather than through groups of people, (it should be noted that while much violence and other issues are related to the misuse of alcohol, most people who imbibe are out to relax and have a good time rather than engage in antisocial behaviour. Also while alcohol use is often maligned in this country in particular, alcohol itself can be a positive social lubricant if taken in appropriate and reasonable quantities). Try to reassure yourself that there is no reason why people in the general public would have any reason to wish harm or have malice towards you in particular. The sense you may have of feeling different or not fitting in does not automatically mean that others in society can sense or see that. People in society are generally well meaning (or in bigger cities in particular — disinterested) rather than having bad intentions.

9 Life expectations with Asperger syndrome *(Stuart Neilson)*

People with autism are plagued by stereotypes of what 'an autistic person' is supposed to be like — from uncommunicative classic autism to single-minded genius. In reality (as autism researcher Francesca Happé says) "when you have met one autistic person, you have met one autistic person" — every person with autism is an individual. Professionals are as guilty as anyone of perpetuating myths of what people with autism are like, and what they are capable of. Common professional stereotypes are that everyone is equally affected by the triad of impairments — lacking 'empathy' (without defining that word), having impaired imagination and being bound by rigid restricted and repetitive behaviours. And yet, when you read books written by people — authors, artists, musicians and animal scientists — they brim with imagination, empathy and escape from conformity.

Public stereotypes often suppose that people with autism are all savants with some special skill, perhaps a skill that must be nurtured to genius status. People with autism are perceived as mathematicians and scientists wedded to pure logic — and therefore they might be prevented from pursuing passions like art or music because those interests might interfere with academic strengths. To any parents reading this, success (in any subject) breeds success (in every subject) — academic achievements are synergistic, building in the most remarkable ways. Children who are taught music from a young age demonstrate stronger mathematics skills than children without music. Allowing students to pursue the subjects they love (in addition to those that are required) will not detract from their achievements. But back to public stereotypes of autistic savants, the truth is that few people are savants. Autism is associated with greater extremes in all kinds of human ability — intelligence, athletic prowess, language — so people with autism are widely spread from poor ability to exceptional, and often have mismatched skill profiles, being excellent at one task and incapable of another (for instance capable of engaging story-telling and unable to plan story-writing).

9.1.1 Bursting some bubbles

'Empathy' must be one of the least-precisely defined and confused terms in describing autism. It is often taken to mean 'capacity for emotion' and yet, even at its simplest, is divided into cognitive and affective empathy. 'Cognitive empathy' is the ability to recognise and respond appropriately to other people's emotional states, and is sometimes taken to be equivalent to 'theory of mind' — on average, people with autism are less skilled at recognizing and responding to emotion in others, and make mistakes leading to inappropriate reactions, or failing to recognize that they are causing boredom or discomfort. 'Affective empathy' is the capacity to feel emotion (including the emotions of others, once correctly identified), and is undiminished in autism. One psychiatrist described this as akin to colour-blindness, where you can see and react to light, and even understand the nuances of colour in complex art, if someone is there to describe and translate for you.

People with autism have imagination, whatever the triad of impairments says. Restrictions in social imagination make it hard to predict how changes and unexpected events (especially those involving people) will change the future. The future is a scary place unless it has been all planned out and made safe, so any kind of change to routine, any unexpected arrival or minor mishap can seem like a major disaster. But a planned future does not need to be simple or routine — it could be the most complex, involving and absorbing of futures that any person is capable of dreaming. Books by and about people with autism show amazing levels of imagination.

I admit that, despite good language skills, I have some social and communication difficulties. I would never make a good 'people-person' or cope in any job involving lots of handshaking, small-talk or networking. But other people with autism do — some are tremendously affable, sociable and socially-active beings who thrive on human contact.

The most pervasive bubble constricting people with autism is that they are all STEM students — STEM being "Science, Technology, Engineering and Mathematics". People with autism, as a group, tend to show higher levels of systematizing and lower levels of emotional distraction — which might both aid STEM achievement — but people come in all shapes. Some do not have those tendencies, and others apply the skills they have in whatever disciplines fire their passions. My greatest passions (outside of mathematics) are poetry and photography. We should not restrict horizons, education, leisure, employment or relationships. We should not drive anyone from studies in the humanities, especially in early school subject choices.

9.1.2 Life trajectories

The image of a life trajectory is very common, a path that people will follow from birth to death, which is frequently an idealised and romantic image. The ideal that many people try to live up to, or think that their parents expect them to live up to, might consist of completing school at school-leaving age, going to college and getting a third-level qualification, finding a first job that leads to a career matching their interests and abilities, marrying, having children and then retiring to watch their own children and grand-children follow similar life trajectories. Few people will match every aspect of the ideal life trajectory, and many of people (possibly the majority) will feel greater or lesser degrees of guilt that they have failed themselves or their parents because their lives have taken a different path.

However, 'normality' in every aspect of life would be a rare form of perfection, and almost every person will differ from the ideal in some or in many respects. People fail some of these idealised targets and still live productive and satisfying lives — and also make their parents proud, even if their parents never say so. Newspapers make a great deal out of statistical findings about changes in Irish society, and some of these popular statistics relate directly to the idealised life. Almost 20% of students do not complete school to Leaving Certificate age, and 50% do not continue to third-level education. 'Unemployment' is a politically-loaded term with various meanings, but about 13% of the working age population is unemployed in the sense of not working and actively seeking work. Overall, including students, people who look after a home and people not seeking work, about 35% of working age Irish people are not in employment. Over 40% of all couples live together before getting married and almost 10% of Irish adults have never married. Somewhere between 3% and 7% of Irish people are attracted to same-sex partners, and sexual orientation can change over a lifespan. More than 30% of children are born to parents who are not married. The number of marriages which end has risen steadily since divorce became possible in 1994, and about 40% of marriages are likely to end in divorce.

9.2 Education, employment and achieving your potential

The single most important change in society over recent decades, the one which over-rides almost everything else, is the disappearance of the concept of a job for life. All people are now expected to find work in imaginative and continuously-changing patterns that are not tied to a single source of income and a single employer. This can be viewed as a positive message that each individual is assessed on the merits of the sets of skills and experiences that they have built and can demonstrate.

A workplace and society that increasingly expects adaptability, flexibility, teamwork and instantaneous responsiveness can be very intimidating for someone with autism. Understanding what personal aspects of your own make-up contribute to unease can be very helpful in identifying suitable life goals and suitable environments. Identifying what aspects of change and flexibility actually contribute to work productivity and efficiency can help you make a case for accommodating your needs to make you personally more productive.

9.2.1 Education

We have written a fair amount about education and do not want to repeat any practical advice here. School days are sometimes spoken of as "the best days of your life" because they are the time when you have no responsibilities (work, children, debts), almost infinite resources (time for almost any subject, and time for leisure) and a glowing future before you. Above anything, your mind is plastic in youth, which means it is able to adapt and conform to almost any learning experience. Learning will never be as easy with increasing age. Learning a fluent, unaccented language is very hard for adults. Unlearning a lifetime of gripping pencils and tools in order to learn how to hold a violin fret is very hard in adulthood.

Whilst you have the resources and opportunities of school and college, it makes a great deal of sense to build a portfolio of demonstrated skills in anything that will maximise your opportunities in later life. Many of the skills will seem useless right now, but society puts great faith in certificates and awards as demonstrations that one individual is more skilful than others at particular tasks. The more of these markers you can collect, the easier life will be later. If your own particular abilities lie outside the normal testing of mainstream schools, then it is possible to develop portfolios (for example drawings, writing and audio or video recordings) or to run societies (for example a cinema club) that record your abilities in a form you can share.

The goal of education is usually seen as maximising employment opportunities, not maximising life opportunities. It is worth visualising where you want to be in the future and what activities or achievements you want in life. Education is when you set up the foundation for later life. An autistic mind can have real difficulties in visualising the future (the worst interview question of all is "where do you see yourself in 10 years' time?"), so it helps to think of practical end goals that you can discuss easily with other people, and work backwards through the intermediate steps that lead towards those end outcomes.

9.2.3 Employment and under-employment

People who are identified as disabled, and people who have had episodes of psychiatric care (such as depression), often find that full-time employment is hard to find or to maintain. Employers have some legal obligation to accommodate disability (only, of course, if you decide to call your autism a disability), but the community and welfare structures that would support both employers and employees to enable continuous, full-time employment simply do not exist in Ireland, or indeed anywhere. Your personal needs will sometimes conflict with the needs of other employees or with changes in work practices, urgent deadlines or (quite simply) with the personality of the new boss. The only way to personally ensure your own rights when an employer does not accommodate your needs, or when you are bullied or harassed at work, is to take some form of legal action through a tribunal or court — which is almost certainly an end to your contract, your relationships with colleagues and future employment in similar areas.

The most appropriate response to this very negative view of employment and autism is greater education, for people with autism and for society. Firstly, this means obtaining the highest level of qualifications and skills you can, because these speak volumes about your abilities. Secondly, this means learning about your own condition and how it affects your ability to perform at your best. Lastly, it means educating society to be more tolerant of the diversity of individual need that everyone has, whether or not they choose a 'disabled' label. A pool of truly gifted and dedicated potential employees is waiting to be tapped by employers willing to accept that some people have extremely mixed skills profiles, complex sensory sensitivities or lives that involve periods of depression or emotional withdrawal.

Some young people finish school and end up in apparently endless cycles of supposed education-to-work schemes that are, in reality, only qualifications for the next level of the scheme. Education-to-work schemes that are supported by employers and involve enhancing the skills for genuine employment are more valuable than schemes designed to reduce the number of 'unemployed' in annual government statistics.

9.3 The "marriage, sex and children" bit

Marriage and children is a set of goals embedded in everything from children's fairy-tales to the curriculum of many third level courses — society expects people to form exclusively monogamous, heterosexual relationships and produce children. Society does not really do what society claims to expect, as the statistics in the introduction to this chapter make clear. Many people rebel against these imposed norms, although most people conform to some or all of them to varying degrees, for at least part of their lives.

The single most important message of this section is that people with autism are sexual beings, just like every one else, who might choose to form relationships and explore sensual experiences or might have no interest in sex. People with autism form lasting sexual relationships, marry and have children — but in order to do any of these things, they must have the opportunity to meet other people and to make their own choices.

9.3.1 Sexuality and orientation

Sexuality is based in part on the biological sexes of male and female, categories that are not absolute — between 1% and 1.7% of people have some degree of intersex, or ambiguous biological sex — but every baby is assigned a gender in which they are raised and to which they are expected to conform. Sexual orientation (the attraction to a particular sex) is not absolute either and about 6% of Irish people identify themselves as being attracted to the same sex, with about 2% of the population identifying themselves as gay or bisexual. The currently-accepted term for describing the diversity of sexuality cultures is "lesbian, gay, bisexual and transgendered" (LGBT).

In addition to this, many people choose not to enter into cohabiting relationships of any form. About 45% of Irish adults are single and about 12% remain single throughout life (based on official concepts of ever- and never-married). Some of these single people are asexual, showing no interest or little interest in any form of sexual relationship. Asexuality seems to be more frequent amongst people on the autism spectrum, but it is not clear whether this is through lack of opportunity, negative early experiences or the imposition of expectations of asexuality by parents and carers. Whilst we should never reject anyone's assertion that they are asexual, we also should not accept it too readily, should never enforce it and should not limit relationships.

Sexuality and orientation are not fixed, lifelong characteristics and many people will experience changes in expectations and preferences in different stages of life. Someone may suddenly discover sexuality far later than peers, lose interest in sex or change in sexual orientation.

9.3.2 Expressing sexuality

Starting with the thing that life throws at you first, sex is both the most exciting and the most terrifying thing that can happen to you. Good sex is one of the most satisfying experiences anyone could have, and the closest that you will ever feel to another human being. Bad sex (especially non-consensual or coercive sex) will live in your memory for the rest of your life, possibly affecting every future attempt at intimacy. Sex is not compulsory — one definition of sexual health is "the sex that you want, including none, without risk of harm" — and a large minority of the population never form lasting sexual relationships. People with autism may have a distinct disadvantage in understanding sexuality and sexual orientation, because having fewer and less equal social relationships means having less opportunity to discuss and resolve such complex issues. If you do feel sexual pleasure and want to have a sexual relationship, then it is necessary to create the opportunities to meet people with whom it would be possible to have a relationship. This will involve social activities, education, your place of worship or people you meet through employment. Relationships develop when there is time for socialising or leisure and when there is time to express mutual interest.

Sex has particular issues for some people with autism because of the immersion in strong sensory exposures — sex is one of the few activities that engage all five senses (sight, touch, odour, taste and hearing) at the same time. Eating is the only other common activity with a similar exposure, although activities like pottery or painting can engage all senses to some degree. You may have to negotiate with your partner how you experience this battery of exposures in a positive way.

Being in some sense 'disabled' by autism will almost definitely mean that family and other significant people in your life will throw metaphorical protective arms around you over issues like love, sex and marriage. Infantilization is the process of perceiving a disabled person as a baby incapable of adult decision-making, in some or all aspects of mature life. If you have not been declared mentally incompetent, then nobody can forcibly prevent you from forming legal adult relationships. Having said as much about your rights to self-determination, I should also say that some of the happiest and most stable couples I have ever met were formed through arranged marriages, with partners chosen by their parents. There is no rational reason why two horny teenagers should be better at judging a good life partnership than their own parents, or other adults who are not driven by hormonal urges.

9.3.3 Children and the genetics of autism

One issue that may arise when you have a diagnosis of autism is the genetic component of the condition, and whether your children would be affected. The simple answer is that the risk is greater, but most people with autism do not have a family history of autism — as the National Institute for Health puts it: *"In families with one child with ASD, the risk of having a second child with the disorder is approximately 5 percent, or one in 20. This is greater than the risk for the general population."* (from www.ninds.nih.gov/disorders/ autism/ detail_autism.htm). This can inform your decision about whether to have children, or when, or with whom (because the chances of a child with autism would be higher again if both parents have a diagnosis). But it can do no more than inform — autism is more likely in your children, but most children will not have autism. There is also a large argument about whether autism should be seen as a bad thing in any case, and whether autism in children should be described as 'risk' in negative terms. It would be wise to resolve this issue for yourself, if it is something that concerns you, before entering a relationship that might involve having children.

9.4 Fulfilment

Fulfilment is often spoken of in vague terms like 'happiness', rather than concrete, achievable actions. Sometimes it helps to think in terms of well-defined milestones like picking vegetables that you grew yourself, looking at your own painting on a wall, seeing your essay printed out or counting the number of friends you have.

9.4.1 Artistic and aesthetic satisfaction

We have covered a lot of these subjects throughout this book, concentrating on the practical steps that will help achieve certain goals, such as studying, going to college and finding a job. All people are victims of the same set of social ideals that life will follow a particular trajectory of education, a job, marriage, children and a career. However, almost every autobiography written by people who have experienced a full life will contain a message that they wish they had done something differently, such as getting qualified younger, spending less time in the office, spending more time travelling or getting to meet people for pleasure instead of work.

In older times, and especially ancient Indian, Greek or Roman cultures, a great value was placed on polymathematism — learning many skills, including life skills and aesthetic skills. Students were encouraged to be proficient in music, poetry and dance as well as with logic, words and numbers. There was greater interest in developing well-rounded individuals during the European renaissance than there is now — but education then was the privilege of the wealthy and not the right of every child. Universal education almost requires that everyone sits behind a desk following production-line paths to employability. There is a great sense of satisfaction in listening to music and being able to play music, to look at art and being able to paint or draw, or to watching a stage play or film and being able to read a play. Some proficiency at these skills helps to understand and enjoy the experience of aesthetic experience, and does not require that you be good at them.

More importantly, skills are synergistic — they work together to enhance each other. As the old proverb says, "All work and no play makes Jack a dull boy, All play and no work makes Jack a mere toy." Some parents and teachers believe that children have a limited capacity to learn, and prevent them from pursuing some subjects like playing a musical instrument or learning an additional foreign language (especially if the child is a 'problem child'). In reality, skills often enhance and complement other, often quite different, skills. Computer programming (for example) has many 'good' answers and some solutions that look wrong even though they work — code is poetry, and good codes looks good and feels satisfying. A written abstract has to convey the essence of a longer text, briefly, but an excellent abstract is like extracting the motif from a musical melody. Looking at an issue in another language often brings surprising insights because, as another old proverb says, "a person who speaks two languages lives two lives."

There is a strong stereotype that people with autism are good with numbers, or technology, or science. This is despite plenty of autobiographical works and testimony demonstrating lives with an incredible affinity for animals (Temple Grandin and Dawn Prince-Hughes), art (Michael Madore, Peter Myers, Gilles Tréhin and Steven Wiltshire), music (Gary Numan, Ladyhawke, also known as Pip Brown, and Craig Nicholls) or acting (Dan Aykroyd, Paddy Considine and Daryl Hannah). The traditional triad of impairments includes "a lack of social imagination", often expressed as an inability to predict how situations involving people will proceed. It is not remotely a general "lack of imagination". There is a real danger that someone with an autism spectrum diagnosis will be nudged into mathematical and scientific pursuits at the expense of the arts, because every mathematical ability will be noticed and artistic or linguistic skills will be ignored.

Every person should use the enthusiasm of youth, along with the proficiency of the young mind to learn new things, to maximise proficiency in every skill that will later be useful to use. Income and productivity are important both personally and for society, but are not necessarily a life-goal at all, rather than a means to provide the resources for personal satisfaction. Some people with autism (including me) have a lot of difficulty understanding the idea of personal happiness and have problems understanding the things that people describe as making them happy. Sometimes it can help to replace the word 'happiness' with a range of things like personal productivity and satisfaction. Many life goals are not things related directly to employment and income, but almost all life goals require resources and therefore require that you work to earn enough money to fulfil those goals. In ancient Eastern philosophy these might be regarded as the three life goals leading to the fourth and final goal of liberation. These four goals are called Dharma (righteousness, duty and learning), Artha (the pursuit of wealth), Kama (the satisfaction of desires) and finally Moksha (liberation).

9.4.2 Religion

Having already mentioned it, it is useful to continue with this important aspect of life. Religion is an important experience for a great proportion of the Irish population, and the Irish Catholic Church has an enduring influence on every aspect of life in Ireland, including sport, government and broadcasting. These influences affect everyone, whether or not they are members or believers.

Religion is a source of social contact for many people and offers a safe environment to make contact with people of all ages and social groups. Religious worship provides a sense of certainty and security, possibly even more so with society's increasingly always-on connection to the uncertainties and difficulties of modern technological life. Religious leaders are also perceived by some people to be excellent personal guides through difficult times. Nobody but you can decide how much you involve yourself in religious life and religious beliefs, although individuals and groups will often try hard to influence you. People going through difficult times are particularly vulnerable to a person who is able to promise certainty, truth and security — a number of religious groups make a living preying on the insecurity of teenagers, young people and adults in difficult relationships.

All major world religions are based on sets of truths and moral guides about how individuals should live their lives and how societies should cooperate. Most individuals and societies — including those professing strong religious beliefs — do not follow lives according to their own religious scriptures. Nevertheless religious books are full of useful and practical guides as well as systems of belief and systems of though that are worth learning. A good knowledge of world religion is useful to both devoted religious believers and atheists, as well as all manner of agnostics and non-believers in-between. Religion can also stretch the mind, especially if you tend to require things to be either true or false, not to be inconsistent and not to be promoted by hypocrites. It can be exciting and personally rewarding to examine beliefs that are dubious, mutually incompatible and preached by people who appear to be motivated most strongly by Earthly (and occasionally sinful) rewards.

9.4.3 Social satisfaction

Social satisfaction is one of the hardest parts of life to get right for someone with autism. Everyone craves human recognition and human contact, but human contact always has a price. Early negative experiences of bullying, rejection and social misunderstandings cause some people to withdraw and become more and more socially isolated.

Just as the poet John Donne wrote "No man is an island, entire of itself", every human requires social contact for completeness. It can be a useful exercise to examine specific times when contact with other people have been pleasing or personally productive and to assess what elements made the experience a positive rather than a negative — the maturity of the other people, the type of location, whether you were engaged in a joint activity and how much control you had over the situation. You can then find places and activities that would be able to replicate the circumstances of those positive experiences. Apart from creating the circumstances for positive social experiences, these will also be the social settings that other people like yourself find comfortable and rewarding — which means more opportunity to meet like-minded people and form lasting relationships.

Some settings that can be positive are special interest clubs, from hill-walking to photography, adult education evening courses, employment and further education. The more opportunities that you make for meeting people, the greater the chances that you will find rewarding social contact.

10 Recognizing Asperger syndrome *(Diarmuid Heffernan)*

In the first chapter of this book and at various points throughout we have made reference to the defining diagnostic and critical features of AS. We have made suggestions regarding how to get a clinical diagnosis and the pros and cons of doing so. There may be signs and signposts throughout your life which suggest that you may have an ASD, or your family/friends/partners may have noticed signs that suggest you may have an ASD. In this chapter we will explore the various signs that may have existed and the (non-clinical) ways for you to find out if you may have an ASD. We will also explore ways of talking to a partner, friend etc who might be on the Autism spectrum. It is imperative that we state from the outset that ASDs exist within the spectrum of the human condition, that is to say that the lines between aspects of an individual's life that clinically set them apart from those that do not clinically set them apart are blurred and ambiguous. In reading this chapter you may find some of it applies to you or to your life while more of it does not, this may be an indication of autistic traits rather than of an ASD. We will explore this further in the following section.

10.1 The myth of 'normal'

Despite the constant move towards a homogeneous middle-ground where people behave and dress alike (perpetuated by the mainstream media in particular) there is no single fixed point at which a human being can be accurately described as 'normal'. Factors of nature and nurture, such as family/social, environmental and economic factors work to shape us as individuals and as, or indeed if, we coalesce into society we generally find niches that suit us, where we feel some sense of belonging — even if that belonging is as part of a group on the fringes of society. The veils of civility that hold society together are predicated on a willingness amongst those who share spaces to co-operate with each other on a number of levels. Much of this civility revolves around communication and interaction, and much of this communication and interaction is based on what we may deem 'soft' interaction, for example small talk (we would define 'hard' interactions as those concrete interactions that are necessary in our lives, for example, discussing work projects with colleagues/superiors) . This soft interaction may also include the 'pleasantries' usually expected in social transactions such as in shops etc. This type of interaction is unquestioned and accepted by most people. For most people on the Autism spectrum soft interaction is difficult and many see it as inexplicable and pointless.

So what if you do not fit into the perceived 'norm', if you do not see the point in small talk or the world you see around you does not make sense, if you have fixed obsessional interests, you cannot see where others are coming from, does this mean you may have an ASD? There are a number of features of ASD that tend to be common to most on the spectrum. In describing these features we are not suggesting that by having them it means you have an ASD, rather it means you may have an ASD or indeed it may mean you have similar characteristics to someone with an ASD (human beings all exist on a spectrum anyway regardless of having an ASD or not, some of the issues we have looked at throughout this book are common to all regardless of whether they are positioned on the autism spectrum).

10.2 Developing self-awareness

It is worth saying from the outset that it is difficult to be self-aware. This is a skill that takes time and effort to develop and even then it is never a given. One of the primary ways of developing self-awareness in terms of ASDs is to begin to recognise the external factors that may indicate a difference between you and your family/peers/colleagues etc. One way of beginning to recognise these differences is to diarise them. It may be useful to read this chapter and then begin to look at the questions and discussions contained within as they apply to your life. This may be a starting point for diarising these issues or indeed any others that may be pertinent, and thus begin the process of self-reporting. This may be a useful tool in gaining some degree of objectivity by noting situations and occurrences in your life that might be significant. In the next section we will look at examples of external factors as potential indicators of difference.

10.3 Recognising external factors of ASD

As previously discussed, objectively recognising aspects of ourselves or our personalities as being different to others is a difficult task and requires self-analysis, reflection and thought. If you have already purchased this book then it is likely that you may feel that there are aspects of your life that you are finding difficult or there are ways of interacting with others that have been problematic for you or possibly others have pointed these things out to you. It is not the purpose of this chapter to diagnose you, however the following section will explore some issues that may resonate with you and in doing so may provide a framework for understanding or an impetus for dialogue with those closest to you.

We will begin by posing some questions that you may contemplate or discuss with others. In adulthood have you found it difficult to make or maintain friendships or do you find social interaction difficult? Friendships may be difficult to initiate and difficult to maintain. As with all other human relationships they require work and the ability of both parties to compromise. Social interactions are variable and dependent on context, culture, one's own frame of mind etc. However the lines between enjoying one's own company and being unable to interact with others are reasonably well defined. It is our experience that the overwhelming majority of adults (though not all) with an ASD we are in contact with would wish to have friends and/or relationships, however the difficulties that social interactions pose lead many people with an ASD to isolate themselves and avoid much social contact.

As stated previously, for many people on the autism spectrum one of the most difficult aspects of daily life is the interactions with others and the interpretation of those interactions. For instance, the recognition of friendliness from others and being able to define whether it is just friendliness or indeed friendship. This may occur in shops for example where your local shopkeeper is always very friendly to you, asks you about your day and seems very interested in you overall. However, they are running a business and most probably speak the same way/ask the same questions of almost everyone who enters their premises. There are other potential external factors indicative of difference such as counting how many friends you have (this does not include casual acquaintances that you talk to very infrequently or people you have only spoken to via social media). The ability to define or recognise a friendship is a difficult one as it varies from person to person, group to group or even culture to culture. One defining element of a friendship however is reciprocity. This means that the friendship is based on mutual affection and respect and that both parties actively engage with each other in maintaining the friendship. This means trying to understand the perspective of the other person, being willing to listen as well as speak and being able to compromise. If you find it difficult to engage with others in a reciprocal way or feel friends take advantage of you in any way this may indicate ASD characteristics. There may be some other straightforward questions to ask yourself at this point such as: How often do you avoid social situations? How long is it since you left your apartment/flat/house? (apart from picking up essentials, shopping etc). If you are not in contact with anyone other than through the maintenance of essentials then this may be an indicator of a difficulty for you. It is important for us to mention at this point that there are other conditions which may cause social avoidance, for example schizophrenia or depression. There are many points at which different conditions intersect in terms of how it manifests in individuals. However, throughout this chapter — and this book — we try as much as possible to describe ASD traits, while acknowledging some inevitable commonality with other conditions.

In terms of living in a flat/house etc, have you created a space for yourself to feel comfortable in, where you are in control of the variables — e.g. noise, smells, light etc? A defining feature of ASD for many people (though not all) is sensory difficulties. These difficulties may manifest in terms of experiencing the noises, sounds or smells that are a by-product of contemporary living in an oppressive way. This means that for example the noises of a busy street may become oppressive to the point of causing a meltdown or that the person avoids the areas that create these sensory difficulties even if that is to the detriment of practicalities such as shopping. A significant number of people with an ASD may take note of the exit routes from a building as soon as they enter it as a way of reassuring themselves that there is a way of escape should the experience of being in that space become overwhelming. There are many with an ASD who may find crowds of people too difficult to deal with. This may mean for example being unable to differentiate the voice of one's dining partner in a restaurant from the myriad other voices in that space, or finding the proximity of others as an invasion of their personal/comfortable space.

These sensory issues may also manifest in the home space where noises, smells, certain lights may cause distress for many. For instance, for many people with an ASD their living space (if shared) may be divided along temporal lines with the space becoming their space when others are out, or they may have created their own exclusive spaces within the house the others are not allowed into. Some pertinent questions you may ask yourself in relation to sensory issues are: Do you have negative sensory experiences in certain spaces and if so do they cause you to avoid these spaces or to try to control them where you can? Have you ever had a meltdown where the sensory inputs you are experiencing become so overwhelming that you either have to extricate yourself from a space/situation or that you need to perform an activity to calm yourself — such as talking to yourself, or any repetitive physical activity that calms or reassures you? A considerable number of people with an ASD use repetitive physical activity to reassure or calm themselves in certain situations.

Do you find that you have a routine that you abide to rigidly, or that you find unexpected change in particular may lead to anxiety or even a melt-down for you? Routine represents security, continuity and reassurance for many people. It is generally a positive thing as it allows us to plan, and it serves to mitigate against the many variables inherent in modern living. It may become problematic however dependent on the rigidity to which people may cling to routine, for example if sticking to a routine causes conflict with, or hurt to others then this may be problematic. At this point it is worth looking at your own life and examining whether you have stayed rooted in a routine to the detriment of other aspects of your life or indeed others' lives? Have people seemed angry or upset at your unwillingness to change routine or compromise? If so then it may be worth examining that need for routine. Rigidity in thinking may also manifest in how people see their lives. Some people with an ASD may see their lives unfolding in a particular way and find it very difficult to negotiate the likely changes that everyone experiences in their plans or in how their lives actually unfold. For instance, some people with an ASD may want to do a certain college course as it will lead them to getting a job in an area that they have identified for themselves as being right for them. They may find however that the college course is in fact different from what they had envisaged, or it may be more difficult, the experience of the classroom may be overwhelming or the social aspect of college life beyond their grasp and this may lead to them dropping out of college, becoming 'stuck' and unable to move on as the reality of the course is so far removed from the expectation, or they may expend so much mental and emotional energy in getting through the course that they are left exhausted and empty, unable to contemplate a next step.

If this resonates with you then it may be worth taking a step back and examining the areas in your life which are always problematic and why. Do you experience a gap between how you want or expect life to be and how it actually is? Numerous people with an ASD may find that they are clear in their own mind what they want to do and how to do it, but then experience great difficulty in making that a reality due to the variables inherent in life and the necessity to be adaptable to these variables including the ability to change ones thinking or path. The propensity for many people with ASDs to want to adhere to routine (even if that routine is problematic in terms of their overall lives) may make it difficult to contemplate any change. The level of adherence to routine is variable from person to person but may include some obsessional elements of Obsessive Compulsive Disorder (OCD) or other 'routine' based conditions (in some cases people with an ASD may get a dual diagnosis that includes OCD etc).

The area of relationships may frequently be an indicator of difference. For instance have you ever dated anyone? It has been our experience as stated previously that many people with an ASD may want to have a relationship but are unable to do so due to difficulties initiating or maintaining a relationship. The ability to strike up a conversation with someone you may have a romantic interest in is a skill that requires practice as is the ability to accept rejection as part of the process of trying to find a partner. Some important questions to ask yourself (if you do not have a relationship) are: Would you like to have a relationship? What prevents you from the possibility of having a relationship? If the answers to these questions involve your difficulties with social interaction and/or worries about having to compromise your time/space with others then it may be worth exploring these issues in greater depth with those you trust.

If you are currently in a relationship but find it difficult to compromise on your time/space/interests then this is similarly indicative of an important conversation you may need to have with others. If you find that your partner/spouse seems to get irritated with you or you feel they may be annoyed with you and you cannot understand why, these may similarly be indicators of the need for an evaluation of your interactions (please note that one's partner being annoyed with you on its own is not a potential indicator — rather in combination with other indicators being flagged).

For many people an indicator of difference is the degree to which social anxiety affects their lives. For instance many people are affected by social anxiety to the extent that it affects their ability to function in everyday life. This is not exclusively an autistic trait or a characteristic of an ASD but it is an indicator of difference depending on the degree to which it affects your life and if it is in conjunction with the other indicators mentioned in this section. Some questions that you may reflect on are: Do you worry about what others might say to you if you go outside, or do you worry that you may say or do something that makes you feel or look foolish? Many people with ASDs become very anxious at the thoughts of interacting, shopping, socialising with others or even just leaving their home space. This anxiety may become crippling to the point of preventing them leaving the house. A further manifestation of this anxiety may be that the person tries to visualise or imagine what will happen when they leave their home space, who they might meet and what they might say, people they may pass on the street, what they will say to the person working at the checkout of the supermarket etc. While the ability to plan is an important one it is also important to note that life is not always linear and conducive to pre-planning. Consequently this type of planning often increases anxiety and prevents action. This is especially true of people with ASDs — many of whom have difficulties managing their anxiety.

Having looked at some issues that may be of consequence to your life now, it may be useful for you to look back at your past and explore any potential indicators of difference that may exist there. One of the first ways of doing this is to talk to family/loved ones/partners/friends about your infancy and childhood. Ask parents and older siblings what you were like as a baby and young child. What age did you begin to talk at? How did you interact with your parents and siblings? Were you able to make eye contact? The ability or inability to give eye contact is seen as a key indicator of ASD by many. For people with an ASD it is a difficult proposition with some people reporting the experience of making eye contact as being physically painful and many others questioning the importance of making eye contact.

Given how unreliable subjective memories are, it is best to talk to others about their perception of events that may have occurred to you in your childhood, for instance did you play with other children in the school yard or did you go into one corner of the school yard and look at the ants filing out of the anthill — which you found eminently more fascinating than the other children. A common thread amongst people with an ASD is a fascination with particular topics. This is present in most children but may be an indicator of difference depending on the level of interest you may have had (or still have) with particular subjects and the extent to which you may have talked about them or the extent to which this excluded interest in other subjects. A further indicator which is worth exploring from an adult perspective is whether you had friends at school or even other children that you played with? In our experience many people with an ASD only began to notice their own difference from other children and other children began to notice difference in them from after primary school onwards (though some were as young as six or seven when they noticed this). Were you picked out or picked on for being different in school? Most people with an ASD report being bullied or picked on at school. Much of this was based on being perceived as 'weird', (often because of the persons' perceived lack of interest in friends) or being seen as a 'nerd' or 'swot'. Taken in isolation none of these examples necessarily signify anything other than the fact that children are all different (and potentially cruel). However if all, or some, of these examples resonate with your life as a child then it may be indicative of something other than the usual childhood differences.

Adolescence is a difficult time for everyone. It is a time when human beings are in transition from childhood to adulthood and have to contend with much change, from the riotous uproar of hormones within the body to the yearning desire for independence. It may be interesting to revisit these years (assuming you have left these years) with family, friends etc and look at how both they — and you — saw your life. Similarly to primary school, did you have friends? As stated in the last section secondary school is often the time when people with an ASD notice a difference between themselves and others, or are made to notice the difference by others.

Did you find the subjects you were being taught stimulating? Or did you find that you were only interested in some subjects which you excelled at academically while you failed miserably at the ones you did not find engaging? What was your experience of classrooms — did you find the noises, smells, light overwhelming? Or did you find yourself hiding from other students as a way of coping with the anxiety of having to interact with them? We have encountered people with an ASD who regularly hid in toilets or cloakrooms rather than having to face interacting with other students or traversing the schools public spaces and the dangers they often contained.

10.4 Screening

The various examples we have described above are a loose coalition of the features of ASDs. They are not designed to be an exhaustive list, nor are they designed to be a basis for a self-diagnosis (WrongPlanet.net provide online tests which may be of interest to you as a signpost towards diagnosis, as may Simon Baron-Cohen's AQ test published in Wired magazine and available online at www.wired.com/ wired/ archive/ 9.12/ aqtest.html. Beware, however, of disreputable online sites offering online tests which are generally unreliable and often involve giving them money). The examples are used as a way of recognizing episodes, characteristics or traits that may point towards ASD (some of the indicators may also apply to other conditions which are treatable so it is advisable you seek professional advice). If you feel that all or many of the examples resonate with you then it is worth seeking a clinical diagnosis. Before deciding to seek a diagnosis it may be worth exploring the idea of screening. The purpose of screening may be defined as a way of detecting potential indicators of difference. These in turn may confirm personal suspicions, provide a basis for discussions within a family / with a partner / with a health-care provider, or to develop self-awareness.

Generally the target population for any screening process is significant numbers of asymptomatic, but potentially at risk individuals. This would include people who feel they may be somehow 'different', have social difficulties, have been pointed towards an ASD diagnosis, identify with an on-screen portrayal, or are reading this book, and are wondering what to do next!

The methods of screening are generally straightforward, they are acceptable to patients and staff and can be entirely private and confidential, you do not need to tell anyone you did it, or what the result was. The positive result threshold is generally chosen towards high sensitivity — not to miss potential difference, therefore many people score high, some score high because of autism, some because they are in a particular emotional space that leads to a high score (and will change over time) and some because they have other conditions with similar expression. It is very important to bear in mind that it is NOT a diagnosis, nor even reliable, it is merely a way of exploring the possibility of having an ASD or in discounting the possibility. Therefore a positive result indicates suspicion of ASD (often used in combination with other risk factors) that warrants confirmation, you could then use this to develop discussions with family or a partner, decide to read more about ASD, or visit a doctor to seek a formal diagnosis, the questionnaire could form the basis of a discussion with a doctor, to explain why you are seeking a diagnosis, and what aspects of life are difficult for you. The cost of screening is free (but with risks of accompanying misinformation, poor quality, bias and political agendas of website author if screening is done via the Internet, the introductory text at www.wrongplanet.net/ postt113459.html suggests that you could have ASD even if tests are negative, and there are so many tests now, some unvalidated, that at least one is bound to indicate ASD).

Diagnosis on the other hand is designed to establish the presence or absence of a condition. It is generally targeted towards individuals showing symptoms in order to establish diagnosis, or alternatively asymptomatic individuals with a positive screening test. The methods of testing may be more invasive than screening but may be justifiable as a necessity to establishing a diagnosis. The likelihood of a positive result is based on high specificity (true negatives). In diagnosis more weight is given to accuracy and precision than to patient acceptability. If an individual receives a positive result, it provides a definite diagnosis. Obtaining a diagnosis may be expensive, however these costs may be justified by receiving a definitive diagnosis. For many people, their family or friends play an integral part in the road to exploring a diagnosis. The next section will look at how family or friends may go about broaching the subject of diagnosis/screening with their loved ones.

10.5 Beginning the discussion

The idea of broaching the topic of either screening for an ASD or seeking a diagnosis is an extremely delicate one for family/peers etc if they suspect that someone close to them may have an ASD. The first thing we must say here is that we know of many instances of people getting a diagnosis through subterfuge on the part of families and this has led to either huge difficulties on the part of the person accepting a diagnosis or indeed in many instances outright rejection of the diagnosis and cessation of contact with family. The bottom line is that openness and transparency are the best way to approach the subject. A good way to begin may be to ask the person themselves if they feel that there are particular areas in their lives that they may find difficult, as well as looking at the parts of their lives that they excel at or enjoy. It is worth having a conversation with your loved one/friend around the possibilities of having an ASD and discussing some of the positives that may be attached to it. For instance, getting a diagnosis need not be a negative in that it may give an individual an explanation for the things they find difficult. It may make the social interactions that seemed inexplicable easier to begin to understand. It may explain a sense of everyone else understanding implicit social rules of the world (when in fact many people with an ASD see the world differently rather than aberrantly, there are no implicit social rules rather there are rules that people with ASDs may not see, understand or agree with!), your loved one may also discover that other people with an ASD may share their perspective when previously they may have felt that nobody else did.

Having the conversation with a loved one about how they may find certain aspects of life difficult is never going to be easy. Many factors may play into how the conversation goes for instance what your relationship is like, are you close, are you able to have a personal conversation with the person. It is important to be sensitive, and it is sensible to have the conversation in a calm and rational way rather than in exasperation or in the heat of an argument. How you present the possibility of screening/seeking a diagnosis to someone has implications on how the person may feel if they get a diagnosis. The receipt of a diagnosis does come with a label and many people feel that the label is stigmatising. When discussing this issue with your loved one it is best to look at the label as merely words that explain aspects of life that your loved one may find difficult. We do not think it is necessarily vital to the person's life that they accept the label (it should be said that some people also enthusiastically celebrate their chosen label) but rather they accept that there are things they find difficult and that there are strategies that may make these aspects of life more manageable. Therefore the actual label of ASD is not the important part of getting a diagnosis, it is the fact that it provides an explanation for the things the person may find difficult and it may lead to finding ways of making life more manageable.

If you have the conversation with your loved one and it goes badly — for instance the person reacts with anger towards the suggestion of diagnosis, it is best not to push the subject. In many cases continuing to suggest diagnosis/screening in this situation may push the person further away from actually considering it — and also from you/their family. It may be worth exploring this book and others (as well as some websites) for ways in which you may support or help the person regardless of them having or accepting a diagnosis or not.

10.6 Differential diagnosis

The criteria for the receipt of a diagnosis of an ASD is necessarily a moveable feast in that it is largely based on social factors which are influenced by a variety of variables such as whether you have a job, what your economic circumstances are, what your childhood was like etc. The fluid and evolving nature of who we are as human beings means that we may score differently on diagnostic tests at different times or places in our lives. It is also fair to say that there other diagnosable conditions that may have some similar features as an ASD, such as anxiety disorders, or schizophrenia. Having an ASD may also make it more likely to have other issues, for instance depression. It is important to bear in mind therefore that you/a family member/friend may have difficulties that appear to be associated with an ASD but this is not necessarily the case.

10.7 Public awareness of ASD

There has been an increasing awareness of Autism Spectrum Disorders in the public sphere over the last number of years. This has been evidenced by the increasing numbers of people getting a diagnosis of an ASD as increased awareness is linked to increased likelihood for people to seek diagnosis. The key means by which public awareness has been raised is through popular culture and the increased numbers of movies and television series that either revolve around or feature a character who is said to have an ASD, including for example the character of Sheldon Cooper in "The Big Bang Theory" where ASD is not explicitly mentioned (we describe this in more detail in chapter 13). In many ways the image of people on the autism spectrum has changed radically from the portrayal of autism in movies such as

"Rainman". Many modern representations of people with an ASD are more subtle and nuanced and may be more reflective of the 'real' experiences of those on the autism spectrum. Books have also had an influence on this with a gradual expansion of the canon of books on ASDs to include not just clinical, medicalised books but books written by and for people with ASDs — such as those written by Luke Jackson or Michael John Carley to name two. These books, and others, discuss the experience of being a person with an ASD, rather than describe a set of symptoms as has often been the case with previous books written by neurotypicals about ASDs. The effect of describing being a person with an ASD from the individual's own perspective has had the effect of 'humanising' ASDs in the public consciousness, as opposed to the image of people with an ASD in movies like "Rainman" or various books on the topic which may have had a 'dehumanising' effect on the perspective of ASDs in the public consciousness.

From an Irish perspective there has been very little attention given to ASDs either in terms of research, books or in popular culture generally (there are exceptions to this such as an ASD character in popular soap opera "Fair City") though this seems to be gradually changing in contemporary times. One of the most interesting ways in which the public consciousness was raised about ASDs in Ireland was through a controversial newspaper article by a well-known local columnist whose views in this particular article stirred an angry reaction amongst people with ASDs, parents, families and partners of those with ASDs. The article had an inadvertent importance in the raising of awareness and understanding around ASD in the weeks that followed it — where television, radio and the printed media were inundated with testimonies from people on the autism spectrum or those involved with/related to people with ASDs. Therefore regardless of the controversial nature of the article the net effect was a positive one in bringing ASDs into the public consciousness and perhaps more importantly allowing voices to emerge and describe the pertinent issues in a way that increased understanding of ASDs in the public consciousness.

The reason the raising of public awareness of ASDs is important is — as stated above — to increase understanding of what ASDs are and to understand the experience of a being a person with an ASD. The books, movies and television series that discuss or are related to ASDs in some way, may also provide a platform or starting point for a discussion around ASDs for many people with their families, friends etc (or vice versa). The fact that there are people with an ASD writing books about their experiences also serves to present ASDs in a more positive light. This is not to suggest that there are not difficulties associated with having an ASD but rather to suggest that while there may be difficulties, these do not necessarily have to define you and in most cases there are many positives to having an ASD. The presentation of ASDs in a positive and human way through particular books, movies etc may be a way for people to begin to develop an awareness around their own difficulties as well as being a way for families etc to begin a conversation with their loved ones.

Ultimately, as time has gone by there is increasing understanding and awareness of ASDs. This is a positive for people with ASDs and for society generally. Raised awareness may mean an easier passage through life for younger generations of people with an ASD — as well as older people. Increased awareness may contribute to a decrease in stigma and the possibility of society embracing and harnessing the many positives of people with an ASD. It should be noted that the one (and most pervasive/far reaching) medium where there is still much evidence of lack of understanding and many negative examples of ASDs is on the internet where ill-informed and occasionally hurtful or even malicious material is widely available. There are also plenty of people offering 'cures', dietary and other interventions, as well as theories about causes and cures. It is worthwhile therefore seeking out reputable sites, books etc if you want to become more reliably informed for your own life or for understanding/beginning a discussion with a loved one.

11 The pros and cons of a diagnosis *(Stuart Neilson)*

In this chapter we discuss the positive and negative outcomes of a diagnosis and a label of autism spectrum disorder. It is important to note that (for us, at least) a medical diagnosis relates to obtaining appropriate resources and medical services, and that it is a requirement of the system to be diagnosed and assessed with needs in order to receive appropriate care. We discuss whether autism is a difference or a disability throughout this book, but acknowledge that State-recognized experts use 'disability' as the basis of needs assessments. We discuss the mechanisms of getting a diagnosis in the third section of this chapter. Diagnosis is not automatic and may require considerable effort and some cost — children under five should be assessed by the HSE, people under eighteen might be assessed while they remain in education (resources permitting), and adults will usually need to pay for a private diagnosis. People under eighteen may also seek a private diagnosis due to the inordinate delays (one to two years) in completing assessments of special needs.

There are many things that you may wish to consider when deciding whether or not to seek a diagnosis, such as whether you will experience any stigma or bad treatment because you have a medical condition, whether it will affect your income, your insurance premiums, or even your eligibility for certain jobs or civic responsibilities (such as jury service). You may already have been diagnosed with an autism spectrum disorder (or related diagnoses), and much of the discussion may still be relevant to whether you choose to disclose your diagnosis to different groups of people (such as friends, teachers or an employer). There are many transitions in life where you move between educational settings, between jobs or move home, all of which offer some opportunity to redefine your decisions about how you present yourself and your diagnosis.

As you read this chapter, it may help to imagine two different thought experiments to help you differentiate between diagnosis and labelling, and to help you evaluate the pros and cons of each. These experiments (or real life, if you know real people in similar situations) are:

Experiment 1 involves looking at one toddler who is assessed and diagnosed with an autism spectrum disorder at the earliest opportunity, goes to school using all available special needs provisions, transfers to secondary school as a special needs pupil and again makes use of every accommodation to make a successful application to third level education and employment as an adult protected by legislation prohibiting discrimination against people with disabilities. A different toddler with similar symptoms and behaviour grows up without that diagnosis or label, quite possibly feeling 'different' from other people but without knowing why. We can see both situations having benefits, and both having disadvantages. The undiagnosed toddler will not be singled out or bullied because of a label, but might be bullied because of being 'different'. The diagnosed toddler may understand personal differences better, but may also find that opportunities (for academic achievement, or of social functions) are limited by other people's limited expectations of what a person with autism can do.

Experiment 2 is to imagine that you could move anywhere in Ireland (or the world). After picking the place with the best climate, the best food, the most unattached single people, or the right level of urban-rural development, consider whether you would select the place with the highest proportion of people with diagnosed autism, or the place with the lowest proportion. The place with the highest rate of diagnosis is clearly recognizing autism as an issue, identifying people affected by it and (probably, given that they are bothering to diagnose) doing something helpful in the way of educational resources, employment protection and social supports. But all those benefits come with the price of having to accept the label and then using that label to obtain the benefits. It is possible that the place where diagnosis is rare is a place where diagnosis is irrelevant because society is more tolerant of diversity and provides better educational resources and legal protection to everyone, without requiring that they accept and identify with a diagnostic label. It is also possible that people with autism spectrum disorder in some societies are simply hiding, and nobody cares — we just do not know. We do know that the frequency with which autism is diagnosed varies tremendously between different places, that not all of this variation is a 'real' difference in the underlying rate of autism, and that social and economic factors drive some of this difference.

(You might know people who went to school before the 1990s, when autism was not diagnosed as frequently and Asperger syndrome was hardly ever diagnosed, and they would have a different perspective from a time when most behavioural differences were attributed to a bad attitude, naughtiness and cheek. Likewise, you might know people from parts of the world where autism is rarely diagnosed).

Both these thought experiments should show that being diagnosed provides useful knowledge about yourself from which you can make very practical gains — just like knowing your running speed, your strength or your performance in maths or language tests. A diagnosis differs from these other things in that it is often accompanied by a label, which usually has a negative effect. It would be great to have the diagnosis and personal awareness without the label, and some people do manage that.

11.1 The benefits of diagnosis

The big question to answer about diagnosis is whether, for you, in your circumstances, a diagnosis is beneficial. Everybody will see the answer differently, and that answer will depend on changing circumstances, and will change over the course of your lifetime. An important point to bear in mind is that you are exactly the same person after diagnosis as you were before, and you will continue to be that same person whether or not you are diagnosed. It might help to see a diagnosis as one more tool (or one more certificate) to use whenever using it has any practical benefit, or leave in the toolbox (or drawer) at times when you do not need it. Autism is not itself necessarily a disability — social demands and external factors disable people who are 'different'.

We will state right up front that we believe that having a comprehensive assessment and a professional diagnosis is a good thing for many reasons, discussed below. It is also clear to us that labelling people is almost always a bad thing, which we also discuss below. A diagnosis need not result in a label, although it often does — particularly, for instance, if a child with a diagnosis is treated differently in the classroom, or attends different classes from classmates.

It is also important to note that in Ireland a diagnosis does not automatically entitle a child, adolescent or adult to anything at all — not to therapy, special education, educational accommodations, employment accommodations or social welfare. The relevant law in Ireland is **The Education for Persons with Special Educational Needs Act 2004** statutebook.ie/ 2004/ en/ act/ pub/ 0030/ index.html (often called the EPSEN Act), which works forward from the term 'disability', which is defined within this Act as *"a restriction in the capacity of the person to participate in and benefit from education on account of an enduring physical, sensory, mental health or learning disability, or any other condition which results in a person learning differently from a person without that condition"*. This is broader than and less medical than the definition in the Education Act 1998. Under the EPSEN Act you have a legal right to be assessed, but not to any subsequent resources, although under Article 42 of the Constitution of Ireland, every child is entitled to free appropriate primary education up to the age of eighteen years. An assessment and diagnosis are the most important step towards obtaining whatever resources are available. The Citizens Information Board describes the history and current legislation on rights to educational supports www.citizensinformation.ie/ en/ education/ the_irish_education_system/ constitution_and_education.html.

The implementation of EPSEN has currently been suspended due to the economic downturn. The implemented parts of the act apply to children under the age five and all subsequent phases of implementation were deferred in 2008. Subsequent governments have suspended further implementation and this was announced as a permanent suspension in 2012. An autism bill has been proposed in the Dáil that may revive some aspects of assessment and intervention for people with autism, both in the early years and throughout the lifespan.

You may not consider yourself to be 'disabled' but from the outset, in Irish law, you must identify with a diagnosed condition and accept that the condition has a disabling impact for the purpose of benefiting from educational entitlements. Here we discuss how a diagnosis can help you to access therapy, educational resources, employment accommodations or protections and social welfare benefits. We then discuss some of the negative effects of diagnostic labelling, and how they might be avoided or dealt with.

11.1.1 Early intervention and education

If a child (that is to say someone under the age of eighteen, in school or before school) has symptoms that impair the child's ability to benefit from education, then there are often therapies that can help the child's development. We say 'child' because that is the extent of the legal entitlement in Ireland. Therapies might include occupational therapy, exercise regimes (and associated equipment), a special diet or sensory training. The expense of therapy can be extremely high, but the lifelong benefits are also great, and increase the earlier that therapy is accessed.

Under the terms of the EPSEN Act, the presence of a disability qualifying as a special education need should be identified by the HSE or by a school principal, although a parent has the right to request an assessment. The usual interpretation of the law is that if a 'disability' is impairing the ability of someone under eighteen from learning, then state-funded therapy is appropriate, even beyond primary education. The Citizens Information Board provides current information about pre-school education www.citizensinformation.ie/ en/ education/ pre_school_education_and_childcare/ early_childhood_care_and_education_scheme.html and special educational needs www.citizensinformation.ie/ en/ education/ the_irish_education_system/special_education.html

In an ideal world, every person would receive appropriate therapy for any behavioural or sensory issues that they have without the need for a diagnostic label in advance, but in this world a diagnostic label of 'autism spectrum disorder' is a short-cut to therapy for every other issue that a person may have. A symptom alone, without a diagnostic label, is unlikely to receive attention or resources.

In summary, it seems beneficial to take advantage of the right to an assessment, and to whatever therapy is available, whilst in full-time education and under the age of eighteen. Even getting diagnosed can be difficult and expensive once over the age of eighteen and out of education.

11.1.2 Education and accommodations

There are a range of resources and accommodations that apply whilst in education, although resources vary tremendously across the country and between schools. There is evidence that some schools use their admission procedures for social engineering to minimize special needs resources and discourage special needs applicants, whilst others actively try to attract special needs students in order to increase their special needs budget, further distorting the inequality between schools. The National Council for Special Education has expressed disappointment in 2013 that some schools erect overt barriers, 'soft' barriers or both to prevent or discourage parents from enrolling children with special needs.

The resources that might be available include transcription of notes, the use of a laptop computer or audio recorder, time with a special needs assistant or resource teacher, extra time to complete some assignments or exams and being examined in a separate room free of the noise, smell and other sensory distractions of a full exam hall. The Department of Education and Skills also runs a scheme to provide an extended school year to children with autism, based either in the school or through home-based tuition. Further details of this July Provision are available at www.education.ie/ en/ Parents/ Services/ July-Provision/

When applying for third-level courses, the Disability Access Route to Education (DARE) scheme provides a limited number of places for people with a disability, a specific learning difficulty or a significant ongoing illness. You must apply for this scheme directly through DARE. You can choose to indicate a disability on the Central Applications Office (CAO) form, along with details of ongoing supports that would assist you in your third level studies. The CAO encourages disclosure of a disability, but disclosure is only obligatory if applying through a supplementary admissions route such as DARE. You can, of course, choose not to identify yourself as disabled and, in effect, lose your disability at this point in your life. Details of the DARE scheme are available at www.accesscollege.ie/ dare/ index.php. The Association for Higher Education Access and Disability (Ahead) provides a useful set of current links to support services throughout higher education institutions in Ireland www.ahead.ie/ links.php.

Citizens Information provides an overview with links to detailed information about the third level application procedure, resources and disability support services at www.citizensinformation.ie/ en/ education/ third_level_education/ applying_to_college/ third_level_education_for_students_with_disabilities.html. As with our comments about school resources, it is a requirement that you identify yourself with the label of 'disabled' in order to make use of the resources that are available in third level institutions. It is your own choice whether the benefits of those resources balance out any negative connotations that you or others may have with the term.

11.1.3 Employment

Workplace discrimination is outlawed under the **Employment Equality Acts 1998-2011** www.irishstatutebook.ie/ 1998/ en/ act/ pub/ 0021/ index.html, which apply to behaviour within the workplace and to recruitment. As with education, the law requires that you identify yourself as "a person with a disability" in order to seek equality with other people who do not have that disability (or have some different disability). The Employment Equality Act requires employers to make "reasonable accommodations" to support employees in the workplace, such as re-deployment to more appropriate tasks, flexible working or workplace adaptations. This could be as simple as changing light-bulbs in order to reduce flicker and piercing noises, or locating a desk away from movement and sensory distractions. It could be as complex as purchasing individual software or assistive technology appropriate to your own needs. In the context of the Act, the 'reasonable' nature of an accommodation is determined by the employer within the resources available — one employer may be supportive and keen to develop skills, whilst another may claim that the costs of support are unreasonable and exceed any benefit to the company.

The **Equal Status Acts 2000 to 2012** www.irishstatutebook.ie/ 2012/ en/ act/ pub/ 0041/ index.html applies even more broadly to any person providing or in receipt of any goods or service, including any "service or facility of any nature which is available to the public generally or a section of the public" — that includes employment, education, shopping, paying taxes or even being arrested. All of these circumstances must involve due regard to any disability which is apparent or declared, with 'disability' defined as "a condition or malfunction which results in a person learning differently from a person without the condition or malfunction, or a condition, disease or illness which affects a person's thought processes, perception of reality, emotions or judgement or which results in disturbed behaviour."

As with education, you need to identify yourself with the label in order to benefit from the resources available. Only you can answer whether the benefits of disclosing your diagnosis exceed any negative impact. We discuss the possible negative impacts below.

11.1.4 Social Welfare benefits

Unemployment and under-employment (being employed in part-time or less demanding jobs) are very common for people with an autism spectrum disorder. This can be due to unpredictable changes in the workplace, anxiety, other health problems and a lack of appreciation of the skills that some people hide underneath shyness and poor social skills. The poor economic climate at the time of writing has undoubtedly made everybody's employment prospects worse, and probably amplified these effects. If you have been employed and become unemployed then you will be entitled to Jobseeker's (unemployment) Benefit on the same basis as any other person who has made adequate PRSI contributions.

You may also be entitled to Illness Benefit for short-term disruptions in work or between jobs that are attributable to illness, or to Disability Allowance if you are unable to find or retain work in the longer term because of an identifiable disability. Autism spectrum disorder is not automatically a disabling condition — many people work productively with autism, or work productively given the right working environment and match with their skill set, but finding an appropriate match to your own particular skill set is more challenging than for many people. You may not ordinarily think of yourself as 'disabled', but if may need to accept this label in order to qualify for benefits to which you are entitled when other people's attitudes limit your employment opportunities. Disability Allowance is also a gateway to other benefits including a Free Travel pass, the Household Benefits Scheme (Electricity Allowance and Free Telephone Rental) and some care allowances.

In all cases, a diagnosis and assessment of your own individual capacities and impairments is essential to apply for a benefit. The Department of Social Welfare will require evidence of any disability from a certifying physician, including the original assessment and regular medical certificates from your GP. The Department may also call claimants in for an incapacity assessment by their own assessors.

11.1.5 Adult health needs

We discussed medical issues in detail in Chapter 7, concentrating on issues that are not primarily symptoms of autism, but may be affected by it — such as difficulties in relating to GPs or in discussing emotions. There is no specific provision based on a diagnosis of autism for adults in Ireland, but there are provisions based on assessments of disability or the capacity to work.

Income supports include Illness Benefit when you are sick, but normally work, Disability Allowance if you have a long-term disability and Invalidity Pension if you have worked and are no longer able to. The last two permit limited therapeutic employment without having to sign off the benefit and then back on again whenever your circumstances change, which is now termed Partial Capacity Benefit. If you do not work and are dependent on someone else, that person may qualify for Carer's Benefit or Carer's Allowance. People in receipt of these benefits may also qualify for a Travel Pass and the Household Benefits Scheme.

If your total income is limited, then you may qualify for a Medical Card that will entitle you to GP care, some hospital care and greatly reduced prescription fees. People who regularly have high prescription charges will benefit from the Drugs Payment Scheme.

Citizens Information has a page of links to detailed information about these schemes, which change fairly often and have complex rules of entitlement www.citizensinformation.ie/ en/ health/ health_services_for_people_with_disabilities/ health_services_for_people_with_intellectual_physical_or _sensory_disabilities.html. If you need further advice, then you can make an appointment at a Citizens Information Centre or with the local social welfare office, or through a charity or other support service that you are involved with.

11.1.6 Handling authority situations

Some people (myself included) have occasional problems in situations where most people would be calm and compliant, but sensory overload and unreasonable intrusions by other people conspire to create confusion or conflict. This is often when the person making unreasonable demands is in a position of authority — a Garda, a psychiatrist, a teacher or an airport security officer — but quite incapable of seeing reason. When the situation is combined with noise, an unfamiliar environment and lots of sensory stimulation, my own behaviour can be interpreted as simply disrespectful or as aggressive and threatening. The information that you have a diagnosis on the autism spectrum can be extremely helpful in defusing a potentially embarrassing situation and explaining that you are not a real threat.

A number of organisations provide one-page leaflets explaining the basics of autism for 'first responders' (Gardai, ambulance and security staff) and you can choose one that you think particularly helpful. One issue that is particularly important is that a high level of verbal skills is easily mistaken as a high level of understanding of the situation. This is pointed out well in the UK National Autistic Society Autism Alert card www.autism.org.uk/ Our-services/ Services-for-people-with-autism/ The-autism-alert-card/ Text-of-the-autism-alert-card-in-English-and-Welsh.aspx. Irish Autism Action sell a photo ID card that can be especially useful with security staff www.autismireland.ie/ autism-id-card/.

Carrying one of these items at all times in your wallet can be quite calming because you can tell people that you have autism when you think it might be misunderstood (for instance if you are taken to hospital, or are interviewed by an authority figure), and take the leaflet or card out if they need further confirmation.

11.2 The negative consequences of a diagnosis

Everything is rosy up to this point — we have described a number of services and benefits that might be available to you, subject to resources and subject to your own degree of 'disability' attributable to an autism spectrum disorder. Now we discuss the downside.

11.2.1 Stigma and bullying

All labels tend to be associated with stigma and prejudice. Just as terms like 'spastic' and 'handicapped' have been become associated with playground taunts and bullying, so might terms like 'autistic' or 'Asperger's' be abused. From primary school onwards, using the diagnosis means being separated from peers and going to the resources room or special needs table in the classroom, or being treated differently in queues or busy situations. Children can be very cruel, and children are very quick to pick out the slightest difference or unequal treatment as a pretext for teasing. What starts as gentle teasing or humour can escalate into bullying, and in any case can be intolerable to the person who receives it day-in and day-out from everybody they meet.

Bullying of course occurs in the street, in pubs and in workplaces as well as schools. Identifying yourself as 'disabled' and seeking accommodations as an adult can be a problem when other people do not see the disability that you feel. This can lead to everything from teasing through to a cold atmosphere or outright hostility.

The big question is one of disclosure. This starts from the very earliest years of a parent deciding when it is appropriate to disclose a diagnosis to a child, and whether the child would be better off with or without the knowledge of the diagnosis. In a school it is possible to have different degrees of disclosure — only to the principal, only to the principal and teachers, and so on — without disclosing to everyone in the class or everyone in the school. Most children have their own behaviours and eccentricities that other children will notice, and you need to identify your own unusual behaviours from the perspective of people observing you. (This can be a difficult task, and having a trusted observer, parent or friend tell you honestly is a big help). Then you need to decide if your unusual behaviours and eccentricities are sufficiently unusual that they require some explanation — of course the explanation need not be autism spectrum disorder, but that is the most likely one to use.

Children tend to become less cruel en masse as they develop, but the abuse becomes more extreme and more violent with older bullies. Therefore secondary school playgrounds often have less group bullying than primary school playgrounds, and group bullying is rare in third level education and in employment. Bullying, when it does occur, can be more intense, more hostile and more dangerous. Harassment and stalking are difficult to deal with. So for our purposes, there is a decision of whether to transfer the label each time we move, from primary to secondary school, from school to third level and when entering a new job. Many people who have used special needs resources in school decide not to identify as disabled when applying for third level, and decide not to register with third level support services. Others who did not make use of special education resources in school do the opposite, registering for disability support for the first time in third level. It is a very fluid choice reflecting very different personal circumstances and personal experiences.

11.2.2 Stereotypes

It is also important to ask whether disclosure and labelling create limitations. A student with a diagnostic label might have certain expectations imposed by parents or teachers, such as being good at the science, technology, engineering and maths (STEM) subjects and bad at everything else, because those subjects are assumed to go with the label. Achievement in 'social' subjects like art or language might not be noticed, or not encouraged. Similar assumptions may be more subtle in the workplace, but could equally push an employee into clerical, factual or routine tasks that the employee is neither interested in nor excels at. Other limitations may exist in social settings, curtailing opportunities available to other people in the same circumstances.

11.2.3 Risks of mis-diagnosis of other illnesses

There may be some health risks to having a diagnostic label, especially a lifelong condition. Once you have a label, it is easy (for both yourself and other people) to attribute any unusual symptoms or behaviour to that one label, without exploring what the symptoms might mean or what the behaviour represents for yourself. If anyone starts to behave in a downcast, erratic, aggressive or emotional manner then it would be usual to explore what has changed in that person's life and whether that behaviour represents distress or a difficulty. Once you have been labelled, it is easy to ignore any new, unusual behaviour because it is assumed to be yet another symptom or trait that goes with that label. Even serious psychiatric illness, such as depression or social anxiety, could be missed or misdiagnosed as just another aspect of autism. Even when illness is not serious, it can add considerable distress when people dismiss your unpleasant experiences as "just another symptom" rather than a real change. The important issue here is that **changes** in your behaviour usually indicate something, and you are often the expert in knowing whether your symptoms have changed.

Physical symptoms can also be overlooked — things like stomach aches, headaches or other bodily sensations may indicate stress or they may indicate physical illness. Most often, of course, aches and pains are a part of everyone's life and have no medical significance. However, it is important to be sure that these primary indicators of illness are treated as seriously as if you had no label.

11.2.4 Insurance and financial services

Ireland has an unusual, and possibly unique health system, in which a dominant State-backed insurer (the VHI) effectively regulates the market in health insurance through its competitive influence. In reality, we have a duopoly between the VHI and

Aviva (the former Quinn Insurance) because no other insurers can afford or are willing to risk the Irish insurance market. This market distortion has been reviewed by the European Court of Justice because it is considered to be anti-competitive, so it is possible that the situation will change very substantially if the VHI is forced to compete freely in the future. However, at present, the VHI is obliged to accept all customers on an equal basis and it makes no difference whatsoever to premiums or cover whether you have any diagnoses or previous history of illness. Prior illness makes premiums more expensive and reduces the range of cover in most other countries.

Under the Equal Status Act 2000 www.irishstatutebook.ie/ 2000/ en/ act/ pub/ 0008/ print.html and Equality Act 2004 www.irishstatutebook.ie/ 2004/ en/ act/ pub/ 0024/ print.html it is not acceptable to discriminate against people on grounds of disability, or to provide services to the public in a manner that disadvantages people who are disabled. The acts also cover treatment of employees and, for instance, treatment of employees by their employer's customers. People who provide services and employment must make reasonable accommodation, in fact *"all that is reasonable to accommodate the needs of a person with a disability by providing special treatment or facilities, if without such special treatment or facilities it would be impossible or unduly difficult for the person to avail himself or herself of the service"*. Excessive cost or planning laws (for instance in adapting a historic building) are reasonable grounds for failing to accommodate an individual's needs.

What this means in terms of services like banking, buying car insurance, finding a mortgage and so on, you should be treated entirely on your ability to pay the bills. Nobody should make value judgements about financial risk or unreliability on the basis of your appearance or behaviour, only on appropriate evidence of financial history. If you have a disability (within the terms of the acts), then it is important to be aware of your rights and able to demand that your rights be respected when necessary.

11.2.5 Travel

There is no good reason why travel — either with a companion or alone — should be restricted because of other people's attitudes to a diagnosis of autism, but it is possible and there are anecdotal stories about staff or other passengers causing difficulties for people with autism. Your behaviour may be misinterpreted by bus drivers, airport security staff or others if you have particularly noticeable stimming or unusual speech. People might even question whether you are able to travel alone or have been "using something" (taking drugs or alcohol). Nobody can be refused the use of surface travel within Ireland purely on the grounds of perceptions, although private bus operators might be more likely to discriminate than public operators. A leaflet explaining autism or an ID card that identifies you as somebody with a disability or autism can defuse these difficulties and make travel less stressful (simply possessing the leaflet or card might reduce your stress levels, even if you rarely or never use it).

Air flight is sightly different in that the pilot of an aircraft (and staff reporting concerns to the pilot) have a duty to provide safety and can refuse boarding to anyone perceived to be a risk. It can be particularly useful to have a written document that explains any behaviours that might be perceived as a safety risk when checking in or passing through security.

11.2.6 Personal freedom

Personal freedom to act as an adult and to manage your own affairs is a human right, but one that can be restricted if you are deemed incompetent through a permanent impairment in cognitive skills or a temporary impairment (such as mental illness). The Irish courts can appoint guardians to manage the affairs of people who are not deemed competent and Irish psychiatric hospitals can detain people involuntarily when they are deemed to be a risk to themselves or to others. Detention in a psychiatric hospital is often called 'sectioning', after Section 3 of the UK Mental Health Act 1983.

A prior diagnosis of autism can make a tremendous difference to the interpretation of your behaviour and your emotional reactions if you experience any mental health problems or are assessed by a psychiatrist. Knowing that you have a condition that limits your emotional expression (called 'lack of affect'), or that you have meltdowns due to sensory overload will certainly improve the chances of getting appropriate psychiatric help.

11.2.7 Civil rights and civil responsibilities

Having a diagnosis of autism should not affect your ability to enter into relationships (including sexual relationships), enter employment, vote in any elections you wish to vote in, become a politician, serve on jury panel, enter military service or undertake 'sensitive' employment such as the secret services or other security work.

A diagnosis of autism is also **not** a get-out-of-jail-free card. You are responsible for your own actions, and if you wish to be treated as an adult citizen, then you also undertake to fulfil all the responsibilities of being an adult citizen. You must pay your taxes, serve as a juror even if you don not want to and obey the law (even the rules that are patently absurd). You can become an activist and (within the bounds of the law) voice opposition to things you disagree with and attempt to change them.

11.3 Routes to Diagnosis

This might be a historical fact for many readers, or a dilemma if you suspect that you have an autism spectrum disorder and have not been diagnosed. The main routes to diagnosis are through the HSE early intervention before school, through EPSEN during primary or secondary school, through convoluted processes involving the HSE in adulthood, or by private consultation with a qualified psychiatrist or psychologist.

11.3.1 Autism spectrum disorder, early intervention and EPSEN

It is most unlikely that traits of ASD will be noticed in postnatal follow-up, or even in early child development check-ups, certainly for readers of this book. Some traits might have been noticed in later pre-school years and led to an assessment and diagnosis by the HSE. Alternatively, parents who believe that their child is different can request an evaluation, although the HSE is not obliged to conduct assessments if they do not believe it is necessary. It is much more likely that you would have received a diagnosis under EPSEN during either primary or secondary school, because a teacher or your parents decided that some form of special education provision was appropriate. EPSEN does not provide resources to help with symptoms or specific educational needs unless there is a formal diagnosis and assessment of need — diagnosis always precedes an individual action plan. The government froze the implementation of EPSEN in 2007, at the point where children under five are entitled to an assessment "as soon as practicable". People under eighteen might be assessed, if resources are available.

A private assessment is available to anyone, at any age, at their own expense. If the assessment is conducted by a registered psychiatrist, psychologist or multidisciplinary team, in accordance with the approved criteria for diagnosis, then report can be used to request appropriate support.

11.3.2 Autism spectrum disorder and the HSE

Getting assessed after school can be problematic, particularly if you do not have clear symptoms or a specifically identified need. A need might be identified in third level education if you struggle with some of the issues that other students seem to do with ease naturally, or if a social welfare officer has difficulty placing you in suitable training or employment positions, or if you have difficulties that other people do not seem to have. One big hint here — many people have great difficulty with things like study plans, anxiety over socialising and relationships or dealing with angry bosses, but they are very good at hiding their difficulties and very good at 'switching off' their problems and relaxing at the end of the day. You have a need in this sense if your anxiety, over-sensitivity to noise, poor communication skills or other autistic traits are having a **clinically significant** impact on your social function, education or employment, in comparison with what would be expected for your age and peer-group. Whether or not you agree that autism is a disability, you will need to tolerate the clinical language for the purpose of assessment. If a lecturer, a social welfare officer or your own GP is of the opinion that you would benefit from an assessment, you can ask to be referred to a qualified specialist — usually a psychologist or a psychiatrist, or possibly a mental health team. It is an unfortunate fact of adult life that autism spectrum disorders fall within the remit of psychiatric health, but a fact that you will also have to tolerate within the assessment process. We must note that State-funded assessment of adults is extremely rare and you are unlikely to be referred for an assessment unless you have very significant difficulties, or are in some form of care already.

A further route to diagnosis as an adult is the accidental one, which is surprisingly common. Many people — about a quarter of all adults — experience depression or episodes of anxiety that cause them to seek or to be referred for psychiatric treatment. There is some evidence that people with autism experience higher rates of psychiatric ill-health, possibly because of the pressure of lifelong anxiety. The symptoms of autism have a large overlap with psychiatric conditions including depression (lack of emotional expression, low mood and limited socialization), anxiety, obsessive compulsive disorder (restricted interests) and psychosis (unusual ways of expressing thoughts). This overlap can complicate diagnosis and treatment, or even lead to people with autism being incorrectly treated for a psychiatric condition that they do not have — treatment that will not be effective, and may be harmful because of the side-effects of psychiatric drugs. However, it is possible for an autism spectrum disorder to be recognized during the course of treatment for something else entirely.

As a side-note, if you are not diagnosed and you feel extreme distress, to the point of feel like harming or killing yourself, then you should talk to your GP or attend any regular accident and emergency department where you can explain the ways that you are feeling and request a psychiatric assessment.

11.3.3 Private assessment

Anyone can ask for a consultation with a qualified specialist to seek a diagnosis of autism spectrum disorder. This includes parents who wish to have a prompt assessment of their child's educational needs — the assessment of children currently takes as long as one to two **years** from the time that parents, medical professionals or educators first note that a child may be performing differently from age peers and requires an assessment. This is a consequence of chronic under-resourcing of special educational needs and is unlikely to change in the near future due to the economic downturn. We list some practitioners in the appendix at the end of this book, although you may find recommendations through charities, personal acquaintances and so on.

It is important to be sure that your diagnosis comes from a qualified practitioner in order that the validity of the diagnosis will be accepted by other people and organisations — for instance a national school principal, a third-level institution, an employer or the social welfare office. A psychologist should be a registered member of the Psychological Society of Ireland www.psihq.ie/ and a psychiatrist should be a registered member of the College of Psychiatrists of Ireland www.irishpsychiatry.ie/ Home.aspx. A practitioner who is employed by the HSE and working from the HSE is likely to be acceptable, as long as their correspondence is on HSE-headed letter paper.

11.4 Summary of diagnosis issues

In conclusion, there are several routes to diagnosis, some of them very complicated. Children under five **should** be assessed in school, other people in full time education **might** be assessed and adults will usually have to seek out and pay for an assessment with a registered diagnostician. Being labelled 'on the autistic spectrum' can have many effects far beyond the simple issue of treating a medical symptom and it is for you to decide if you want that label. Only you can decide whether a diagnosis is on balance a helpful or harmful thing for you, and often it will be a compromise between the stigma of a label and the benefits of explaining your eccentricities or obtaining valuable resources.

There are many transitions in most people's lives where you could decide to change aspects of how you present yourself, and how much emphasis to put on your autism. These transition occur when you change school, move home or change job. You could decide to use or lose the diagnosis at many of these, with each new group of people you come into contact with.

12 ASD research and the future (Diarmuid Heffernan)

The defining feature of the discourse around ASDs in contemporary times is a lack of cohesiveness and agreement. The most cursory of internet searches reveals a myriad of sites dedicated to discussion boards, research, diets, interventions and different organisations who are often saying similar things but are divided due to geography or even in some cases have divided because of personal/political differences between members of the organisation. In this chapter we will look at some of the contemporary discourse, explore some of the current research and look at what the future may hold for those with ASDs, ASD traits and their families in Ireland in the coming years.

12.1 The DSM-5 and its implications

The recent publication of the new fifth edition of the Diagnostic and Statistical Manual of Mental Disorders (DSM-5) has created much discussion, debate and controversy. The Manual has changed the criteria for diagnosis of ASD from three main criteria based on the triad of Impairments to two main criteria — in the DSM-IV these were impairments in communication, social interaction and restricted interests and repetitive behaviours, in the new DSM the communication and social interaction criteria are combined based on social/communication difficulties. The new DSM also subsumes autistic disorder, Asperger's disorder, Pervasive Developmental Disorder Not Otherwise Specified (PDD-NOS) and Childhood Disintegration Disorder into one category — Autism Spectrum Disorder (ASD). The other most significant aspects of the Manual are a recognition of the fact that while most individuals with an ASD will have symptoms in childhood — many will not have difficulties until later in life and this will now be taken into account when people are seeking diagnosis.

The new Manual has appeared in trials to be more accurate in its diagnosis of ASD than its predecessor. It also seeks to address the ethnic and socio-economic imbalance in terms of diagnosis given that the predominant population of people diagnosed with ASD heretofore has been middle class white males, while other ethnicities and socio-economic groups have tended to remain under-diagnosed or diagnosed with PDD-NOS.

There is however much disagreement on the new criteria from a number of different perspectives. Primarily the lack of consensus revolves around the decision to subsume sub-categories of ASD into one inclusive category. For many people this simultaneously denies individuals with Asperger syndrome, for example, their own separate identity and also potentially allows people who do not meet the new slightly stricter criteria to remain undiagnosed but symptomatically on the fringes of ASD. Given that ASDs exist within a dimensional framework, that is to say that individuals on the autism spectrum have more extreme versions of the same traits as most people throughout the population have, it could be argued that the differences between being diagnosed with a Social Deficit Disorder as opposed to an ASD may be the difference between receiving support or services — or not. The new DSM also has implications for many who have already received a diagnosis of Asperger syndrome, high functioning autism etc in terms of whether they will need to be re-assessed in order to meet criteria for supports.

As many people with an ASD have received their diagnosis in adulthood, this has required much adjustment on their part and on the part of their families, spouses etc. For many of the people in this category, the diagnosis represents an explanation of the difficulties they may have experienced for many years and a recognition of the fact that they were not alone. In fact for many it may mean being part of a community for the first time in their lives and this may give them an opportunity to have an identity based on the way they are as opposed to the way many felt they should be. The subsuming of the different categories into ASD in the new DSM in many ways serves to take away that specific identity and categorise people in a spectrum that contains huge differences and in doing so it seems to deny the heterogeneity of the autism spectrum.

A further criticism of the Manual from many commentators is its links with the Pharmaceutical industry and how the new manual has (outside of ASD) created many new categories of disorder which may need to be medicated (we will come back to the topic of medicalisation later in this chapter). Simon-Baron Cohen and others have criticised the new Manual because of (amongst other things) the difficulties it will cause for research of ASDs given the heterogeneity of individuals on the autism spectrum. In the next section we will look at ASD research in contemporary times.

12.2 ASD research — money and medicalisation?

Much of the contemporary research around ASDs seems to revolve around notions of causation and cure. Much of the 'cure' in this research seems to involve medication and is rooted in a 'medical model' philosophy which places the responsibility for disorder or disability firmly in the hands of the individual 'afflicted'. It also emphasises notions of 'cure' of an individual's seeming aberrance as opposed to promoting acceptance of difference. There are many drivers behind this type of research including powerful autism lobbying groups who have sufficient funding to carry out new research. This is not to suggest that all research is cure-based but rather that it is the research that appears most prominent currently.

The other significant aspect of contemporary research is the variety of theories regarding ASD. Some examples of this are a research paper from 2001 which suggests the possibility of ASD being an evolutionary modification by the human brain to the technological age, while a paper from 2011 suggests that the traits of ASDs are remnants from an ancient way of life. This (2011) theory proposes that some of the genes that contribute to ASDs may have been selected and maintained due to the benefits they brought to a hunter gatherer who may need to forage alone for food, and may need to perform repetitive activities.

A common feature of the vast majority of modern research around ASDs is that it is being carried out by scientists, medical professionals etc who are neurotypical. It is an 'outside looking in' approach to ASD and is predicated on a medicalised view of the condition as a disease. This is not to say that research is not being done by scientists etc in collaboration with individuals with ASDs, or that people with ASDs are not writing articles/books from their own perspective, rather it is to say that contemporary research seems to be more focused on causes and cures rather than the experience of living with an ASD or indeed the experience of having a distinct ASD identity in a world largely run by neurotypicals. A final example of this type of medicalised research is in an article from a research journal in 2001, which studied the effects of teaching children diagnosed with an ASD to imitate others (and thus behave 'normally') as a way of preventing the development of their autism.

12.3 Genetics and heritability

What does seem to be emerging from the research in general is that there is a genetic component to ASDs though this has not been narrowed down beyond an array of genes that may influence whether an individual has an ASD or not, and may still be predicated on environmental factors. A particular focus for modern research has been on protein synthesis in the brain and whether the manipulation of the mechanisms of the brain cells may influence 'autistic' behaviour. In fact one study has explored this topic and looked at the potential for pharmacological intervention in changing this behaviour. Research into the heritability of autistic traits has shown a high level of heritability. For instance a study carried out in 2005 by Happé et al explored the similarities and differences in autistic traits between monozygotic twins (identical twins, from the same fertilised egg) and dizygotic twins (non-identical twins from two different fertilised eggs). This type of comparison is used as a standard way of determining the genetic basis of a particular condition and in this study showed that if a monozygotic twin had a high or low score on an autistic trait then the high likelihood was that other twin would score the same. There are believed to be specific genetic variations passed on through families which lead to autistic traits and an increased incidence of ASD in these families — known as 'multiplex' families.

This research is complicated, however, by the fact that genetics is not the only component factor in ASD, as it is also possible for someone with no history of ASD in their extended family to have an ASD, this is referred to as 'simplex' autism and is thought to be linked to 'de novo' changes in DNA sequences which is a one off change occurring in the formation of gametes (cells that unite during sexual reproduction to form zygotes). It is estimated that these variants account for approximately ten percent of all people diagnosed with an ASD (NAS, 2013).

12.4 MRI and brain imaging

The use of brain imaging and particularly the use of magnetic resonance imaging (MRI) has been increasingly discussed as a way of diagnosing ASDs. Kings College in London have recently developed a technique using a fifteen minute MRI scan to diagnose ASD. The scan analyses and evaluates the structure and shape of the cerebral cortex (the outer layer of the brain) and in tests has been 90% accurate in identifying those already diagnosed with an ASD. The research is significant in that it is the first proven biomarker — given that autism has been diagnosed behaviourally heretofore. The test does not serve as a way of screening for ASD but rather as a way of confirming diagnosis given the potential ambiguity of a behaviourally assessed diagnosis. The diagnosis of ASD will continue unless/until ASD could be diagnosed solely by an MRI scan. At the moment the scan does pose some ethical issues such as: what if an individual had never shown any of the behavioural symptoms of ASD, yet were diagnosed with autism based on a structural difference in their cortex? Overall this research serves to add to the canon of existing research around ASD. It also seems to prove a neuroanatomical difference in ASD and this may have some significance in understanding the causes of ASDs.

12.5 The Autism Bill in Ireland

In line with other countries, Ireland has proposed an Autism Bill which sets out a vision for the support of people with ASDs in this country. The Bill was proposed by TD Michael McCarthy and it closely follows the Autism Act 2009 in the United Kingdom in its content. The main proposals of the bill include a National Autism strategy for services for people with ASDs through the life-cycle, which would be overseen by the Minister for Health and implemented across departments (e.g. the HSE Local authorities etc). The Bill proposes a clear pathway to diagnosis and a plan for support following diagnosis including meeting the needs of people with ASDs in employment, access to services and family support. The plan also proposes staff training in public bodies and a national public awareness campaign. As we write, this Bill is due to be debated in the Dáil and we await the outcome of those debates in terms of a timeframe for this Bill to become and Act and its subsequent implementation (this process took a number of years in the UK).

12.6 ASD — current media and internet discussions

We have previously dealt with various portrayals of ASD in the media through movies, television series etc. However there is also a growing discussion of ASDs on the internet through media articles and through blogs, forums etc, and there are a huge array of perspectives on ASDs. What is emerging from much of this discussion is an increase in interest/comment etc on ASDs and a commensurate increase in speculation around ASDs. This includes speculation on people in the public eye who might have an ASD, people being posthumously 'diagnosed' with an ASD and attributing ASD to people who have been in the news for a variety of reasons in the last number of years. There is, therefore, an emerging duality in the understanding of ASD as presented in the media and internet in that there is increased discourse around ASD but there is also increased speculation around what people with ASD may or may not be capable of doing. In contrast there is much positive online discourse around ASD and many good forums (such as wrongplanet.com) have emerged in the last number of years which provide a platform for people with ASDs to represent themselves publicly. This emergence has provided an invaluable counterpoint to the negativity of some of the discourse as described here previously. It also serves as a platform for people with ASDs generally, where they can express themselves, give opinions and seek advice from peers through reliable forums.

This serves to create a sense of community and allows individuals with an ASD or autistic traits to express their identity as a community.

12.7 ASD and the future

The future for people with ASDs is looking considerably brighter in Ireland and indeed the world than it did ten years ago. The increase in understanding of ASD combined with an increase in the public voice of individuals with an ASD has led to initiatives such as the Autism Bill being debated by the Irish parliament. There is still a long road to be travelled however in terms of the delivery of services and supports for those diagnosed with an ASD. Some of the recent modern discourse around ASDs in Ireland has referred to the condition being an 'epidemic' comparing ASD to the HIV virus in terms of the spreading of the 'disease'. This type of rhetoric does not serve the people who have a diagnosis of ASD well in that it serves to stigmatize the condition and is again rooted in a medicalised cure-based perspective on ASDs. It does not promote the idea of an ASD identity which is equally as valid as a neurotypical identity and it does nothing to promote accepting and indeed embracing difference as being the most inherent of all human characteristics (despite the fact that the notion of 'difference' is packaged as 'individuality' and sold to us on a second-by-second basis as a way of convincing us to buy a variety of products by a variety of companies).

The new Autism Bill provides the promise of a joined up autism strategy which would finally show a recognition by the State for the need to place autism supports/needs etc on a statutory footing. We hope at this remove that the Bill and the subsequent strategy do not prove to be yet more rhetoric on the provision of rights (for example please refer to the Disability Act which — though much heralded — merely provided a statutory right to a needs assessment but nothing more than this!).

In the coming years it is likely that there will also be an increasing emphasis on the diagnosis and 'treatment' of children with ASDs. While it is inevitable that this will become a focus of the discourse around ASD it does not deal with the experiences of those adults who are recently diagnosed or not yet diagnosed. The historic treatment of adults with an ASD in this country and others has been damaging both to the definitions of rights and citizenship that most countries adhere to, and to the individuals who have had these experiences. It is positive to note that despite the fact that these experiences cannot be undone, and that this State and this society still have a considerable distance to travel in terms of accepting and supporting people with ASDs, we have come a long way from the dark days where people with ASDs were misunderstood, misdiagnosed and often shut away because they were deemed to be untreatable. A brighter day now beckons.

Appendices   Further reading and resources *(Stuart Neilson)*

These appendices provide information about further resources, websites and the contact details for various organisations and services. I can never hope to be consistently up-to-date in such a vast and ever-changing field, so nothing here can be considered as an endorsement, but many of the details are my own opinion or are recommendations of people who have used a book or service and found it helpful.

Appendix A is a collection of brief personal reviews of depictions of autism is films, on TV, in popular fiction and in factual accounts such as news reports.

Appendix B lists a collection of books that cover (in much greater depth) the topics in this book, a collection of books that are written by people who have a diagnosis on the autism spectrum and a list of websites and discussion groups about autism. The websites were active at the time of publication.

Appendix C is a list of useful addresses of organisations and individuals who provide services for people with autism, with a focus towards the adolescent and adult age range — the audience that this book is aimed at.

Appendix D is a glossary providing a brief explanation of technical terms and acronyms that appear in the text. Some explanations include a link to a relevant website.

A   Autism in fiction and the media *(Stuart Neilson)*

This is a collection of short descriptions of films, books and other references to people with autism in popular media. All the characters are either grown up, or children in situations that an adult might be able to relate to their own circumstances — for instance representing their own fears of social situations, or the fear of losing of control. The collection all portray real-life situations in which you may find yourself, or imaginary situations that can relate to real life — nobody is as intellectually-gifted as Dr Spencer Reid, but we can all relate to the situations involving team membership or relationship problems. Films and books can be a way of discussing situations in a safe or comfortable setting.

The characters are not intended to represent real people with autism as a group, but a diverse group of very individual people who also have autism. Watching the film or recommending the book to a family member, friend or lover may be an opening to discussions about how you and the character are alike and dissimilar. Likewise, the situations portrayed may help explain the way that you feel about similar (or totally unrelated) situations — for instance the recurring themes of being dealt with by authority figures, managing public transport or the difficult-to-explain fear of social and public places.

None of the films are chosen as "explanations" of what autism is, no cutesy or heroic characters feature and all the films are chosen because they represent the perspective of the character with autism.

The film "Rain Man" is included because it remains the best-known reference point for autism, and because many people believe all people with autism are like Raymond "Ray" Babbitt.

Above all, one or more of the characters or films might be your personal role model, or represent a lifestyle that you aspire to. One interesting feature throughout many of these portrayals is how imaginative and empathetic the characters with autism can be.

A.1 Films

Hollywood and national films have tried to portray people with autism with varying degrees of success, and the number of films with characters who are explicitly stated to have autism has risen tremendously in the last decade. It is really worth noting that not one of these films was made by actors with autism, so they are all interpretations of autistic behaviour. The classic Rain Man remains the best known film. Our brief descriptions only name principal characters who have autism, unless another character especially warrants a name-check, because we are interested in whose perspective is being portrayed and how positive the portrayal is.

"Adam" (2009) Adam Raki is a young man with autism who lives with his father. After the death of his father, Adam Raki (Hugh Dancy) finds himself living alone. The film follows his touchingly inept courtship of a beautiful neighbour and the ups and downs of their romance. Hugh Dancy's intense preparation for the role, under the guidance of trained autism counsellors, shows in a convincing portrayal of a young adult with autism.

"Barfi!" (2012) A turbulent Bollywood love-triangle involving a likeable deaf-mute troublemaker and his lifelong relationships with an unhappily married woman and with his childhood friend with autism, Jhilmil Chatterjee (Priyanka Chopra).

"Ben X" (2007) Not to be confused with the American cartoon "Ben Ten", this Dutch film portrays teenager Ben (Greg Timmermans), who has autism. Ben retreats from vicious bullying into a world of multiplayer video gaming, and then contemplates suicide. A fellow-gameplayer encourages him to be as brave in real life as he is in virtual life. It is based on the novel **"Nothing Was All He Said"** by director Nic Balthazar. The title is a wordplay on the Dutch *"ik ben niks"* which means *"I am nothing"* in English.

"The Black Balloon" (2008) Charlie Mollison (Luke Ford) is a teenager with autism, whose younger brother is struggling with adolescence, sexuality and conformity, all compounded by his own resentment of Charlie's behaviour. Ultimately he, and the family, show an uncompromising acceptance of Charlie.

"The Boy who could Fly" (1986) Eric Gibb (Jay Underwood) is a teenager with autism who has never spoken. Orphaned by a plane accident, he is convinced that he can fly and could have saved his parents. His recently-bereaved neighbour gradually gains his confidence and shares his dreams.

"i am sam" (2001) Sam Dawson (Sean Penn) is a single father who has been diagnosed with *"autistic tendencies and mental retardation"* who loses custody of his daughter because he is not competent to assist her learning, but battles to retain his relationship with her as she grows up.

"Extremely Loud and Incredibly Close" (2011) Oskar Schell (Thomas Horn) is a boy with Asperger syndrome who tries to solve a puzzle left by his father, who died in the 9/11 terrorist attack on the World Trade Center. He says that he has been tested for Asperger syndrome, which his Dad said is "for people who are smarter than everybody else but can't run straight". His autism-related fears and difficulties oblige him to seek help from family members, changing his relationship with them and with his environment. It is based on the novel **"Extremely Loud and Incredibly Close"** (2005) by Jonathan Safran Foer, although the novel itself makes no reference to autism.

"Mary and Max" (2009) This is a beautiful, madcap animation featuring New Yorker Max Horovitz (voice of Philip Seymour Hoffman), a Jewish man with autism who lives alone. Max is accidentally drawn into the world of a lonely 8-year-old Australian girl who randomly selects him as a penpal. A lifelong correspondence follows, with humour and some sad interludes.

"Mercury Rising" (1998) This action-thriller portrays a more stereotypical child with autism, the mathematical genius Simon Lynch (Miko Hughes) who has a meltdown when strangers touch him, or when his routine is disrupted. It does portray an exceptionally sensitive understanding of the boy's needs by a stranger, FBI agent Art Jeffries (Bruce Willis). Based on the novel **"Simple Simon"** (1996) by Ryne Douglas Pearson.

"Mozart and the Whale" (2005) This is a love story featuring two characters with autism, Donald Morton (Josh Hartnett) and

Isabelle Sorenson (Radha Mitchell). Donald Morton falls for Isabelle Sorenson when she attends a self-help group that he coordinates, and they have to navigate the jealousies within the group and their own personal difficulties in the relationship. Isabelle Sorenson also has some serious psychiatric issues that affect her ability to commit to a relationship.

"My Name is Khan" (2010) is an epic story of a muslim boy called Rizwan Khan (Shahrukh Khan) who is diagnosed with Asperger syndrome. He moves to America, marries and settles down. His world is overturned by anti-muslim prejudice when his son dies in a beating at school, because his name is Khan. Rizwan Khan determines to tell the US President that "My name is Khan, and I am not a terrorist".

"Rain Man" (1988) The story of Raymond "Ray" Babbit (Dustin Hoffman) is the most-quoted of all films about autism, and the term "Rain Man" is now becoming common in hip-hop and rap music — the term 'rainman' originally meant a trader who brought in successful deals. Raymond "Ray" Babbit is an idiot savant, a socially-inept mathematical genius whose character is a composite of a number of different real people, principally Kim Peek. It is noteworthy that Kim Peek probably had FG syndrome, an X-linked syndrome that mimics autism.

"Salmon Fishing in the Yemen" (2011) is the story of a crazy scheme to bring Scottish salmon-fishing to the desert in the Yemen. Fisheries expert and civil servant Alfred Jones (Ewan McGregor) reluctantly agrees to collaborate, after pressure from on government officials to create a good news story about the Middle East. A colleague complains that *"anyone who, frankly, wasn't suffering from some kind of Asperger's"* would have shown more sensitivity to her feelings, when he reveals that he does in fact have Asperger syndrome. The film is also a complicated love story.

"Snowcake" (2006) follows a man who was the driver in an accident that results in the death of the only daughter of Linda Freeman (Sigourney Weaver). Linda is a woman with autism who lives alone by choice. The driver feels an insatiable need to seek forgiveness from Linda Freeman, whose attitude to the death and his feelings both puzzle and enrage him. His presence in a close-knit rural community draws attention, but also changes the way that Linda Freeman interacts with her neighbours. Sigourney Weaver delivers a convincing performance of an adult with severe autism.

"Temple Grandin" (2010) is a biopic of the animal-handling expert and autism advocate Temple Grandin (Claire Danes and Jenna Hughes), who was diagnosed with autism at the age of two. She is a professor and has a PhD in animal science. Temple Grandin also starred (as herself) in the BAFTA-winning animated documentary **"A Is for Autism" (1992)**, **"Horse Boy" (2009)**, **"When Animals Adopt" (2011)**, the mystery **"The Being Experience" (2013)** and the US TV series **"Animal Odd Couples" (2012–)**.

"What's eating Gilbert Grape" (1993) A film about events around the eighteenth birthday of Arnie Grape (Leonardo DiCaprio), who delivers a reasonably innocent performance of a teenager with autism. The feelings of his older brother and carer, played by Johnny Depp, receive more prominence.

A.2 TV

These are television series set in Ireland or available to Irish viewers in which a character with autism is featured with any prominence.

"All Saints" is an Australian TV hospital drama. It presented the architect Theo Wellburn (in the episode "The hand you're dealt") as skilled, loyal and socially inept. Theo Wellburn rejects the diagnosis of Asperger Syndrome. Dr Frank Campion (the head of the emergency room) has a daughter Kathleen with autism. She frequently features in the series, but Kathleen's perspective is rarely presented — the most frequent issue is which of her professional parents can spare the time and resources to care for her.

"The Big Bang Theory" is a US TV comedy series. Despite many claims that Dr Sheldon Cooper has Asperger syndrome, the show's co-creator Bill Prady has consistently stated that Sheldon's mother never got a diagnosis. The show revolves around a group of nerdy PhDs (including one woman, Amy) and their interactions with young women. The majority of the principal characters are socially inept, which provides many opportunities to explore social norms and expectations.

"Criminal Minds" portrays the character Dr Spencer Reid (Matthew Gray Gubler) as a genius with autism who has a photographic memory. Matthew Gray Gubler said that he plays Dr Spencer Reid as *"an eccentric genius, with hints of schizophrenia and minor autism, Asperger's Syndrome. Reid is 24, 25 years old with three Ph.D.s and one can not usually achieve that without some form of autism."* Reid works in a supportive team and experiences a range of realistic life challenges.

"Fair City" is an RTE soap featuring a physiotherapist called Robert Daly (Sam Peter Corry), who has Asperger syndrome, and his relationships.

"Home and Away" is an Australian soap that once featured Mikey Dunn (Trent Atkinson), an adult with autism, and later Brendan Austin (Kane O'Keeffe), an adolescent with autism. Both roles featured the impact of autism on the family and others, mostly as a challenge that other family members rose to. Brendan is portrayed as growing more independent and self-sufficient.

"Shortland Street" is a New Zealand soap featuring head of surgery Dr Gabrielle Jacobs (Virginie Le Brun), who has Asperger syndrome, her professional relationships and her on-off love-life.

Skins is a British teen drama series from E4 which features Jonah Jeremiah "JJ" Jones, a socially inept teenager with Asperger syndrome whose friends are alternately amused and irritated by him. His social confidence and autonomy progresses over the first four series, in which he features.

St Elsewhere features a minor character called Tommy Westphall (Chad Allen), who takes on a greater significance in the final moments of the last episode of the 5-year run when Tommy Westphall's father asks *"I don't understand this autism. I talk to my boy, but I'm not even sure if he ever hears me. Tommy's locked* *inside his own world. Staring at that toy all day long. What does he think about?"* The toy is revealed to be a snowglobe containing a model of St Eligius, raising the possibility that the entire St Elsewhere universe exists only in Tommy Westphall's mind.

"The Undateables" is a Channel 4 reality series about people with challenging conditions (who the show claims are often considered 'undateable') attempting to find love. Richard, a 37-year-old amateur radio enthusiast, features in episodes 1 and 4 of series 1. Heather, a 38-year-old who also has OCD, features in episode 4 of series 2. As with all reality TV, it both raises awareness and exposes the privacy of the (real) people featured in it — it is not sensationalist and does not ridicule them by the standards of most reality TV.

A.3 Books

These are fictional books in which one of the lead characters is either explicitly stated to be have autism, or in which other characters believe the character to have autism.

"The Curious Incident of the Dog in the Night-Time" (2003) by Mark Haddon uses the death of a poodle, investigated by 15-year-old Christopher John Francis Boone, *"a mathematician with some behavioural difficulties"*, to explore family relationships and the world from the perspective of an outsider. The story is told in the first person by Christopher John Francis Boone, often describing both his own inner feelings and the effect that his outward behaviour has on other people. Mark Haddon has said and written that he is not an expert and that *"curious incident is not a book about Asperger's. It's a novel whose central character describes himself as 'a mathematician with some behavioural difficulties' ... Labels say nothing about a person. They say only how the rest of us categorise that person. Good literature is always about peeling labels off. And treating real people with dignity is always about peeling the labels off. A diagnosis may lead to practical help. But genuinely understanding another human being involves talking and listening to them and finding out what makes them an individual, not what makes them part of a group."*

"The Girl with the Dragon Tattoo" (2005) by Stieg Larsson
portrays a complex young woman called Lisbeth Salander, who is
a talented information analyst, investigator and computer hacker
with limited social skills. Lisbeth Salander has a strong sense of
morality and justice that often brings her into conflict with society's
rules. Lisbeth Salander's journalist colleague and her guardian
believe she *"has Asperger's, or something like it"*, whilst her doctor
and her psychiatrist say that she has *"Asperger's syndrome ...
some form of autism ... is almost autistic"*. Lisbeth Salander
herself refuses absolutely to submit to any form of assessment by
a system that she perceives as hostile and intrusive, so she has
no formal asessment or diagnosis. The author Stieg Larsson died
before revealing his own influences in writing the character.
Lisbeth's conflicts with the Swedish authorities and her evolving
diagnosis are revealed further in **"The Girl Who Played with
Fire" (2006)** and **"The Girl Who Kicked the Hornets' Nest"
(2007)**.

House Rules (2010) by Jodi Picoult follows the investigation of
Jacob Hunt, an 18-year-old with Asperger syndrome who is
accused of murdering his social skills teacher. Jacob Hunt has an
obsessive interest in details and a strong sense of order.

The Rosie Project (2012) by Graeme Simsion is the story of
Don Tillman, a genetics professor who (unknown to himself) has
Asperger syndrome, despite teaching about the condition. The
story follows his dedicated pursuit of social and romantic
relationships, which he initially structures as formal scientific
processes.

A.4 Real life

A number of real-life characters appear in news items and in
popular culture. To the extent that we do not know them, or read
their non-fiction writing, we predominantly read stories about them
that present an image rather than reality. These images are also
used as either ideal models or as stereotypes of autism, some of
which are helpful and many of which can be unhelpful
comparisons.

The computer hackers **Ryan Cleary** (a British LulzSec who accessed servers operated by the CIA and the Pentagon), **Adrian Lamo** (an American hacker-turned-security-expert who exposed Bradley Manning) and **Gary McKinnon** (British hacker responsible for "the largest military hack of all time" searching for evidence that US organisations had suppressed the truth about UFOs, amongst other conspiracies) have created colourful headlines and moving personal stories. The ultimate failures of extradition requests and legal proceedings have underlined the problems of conflicts between public morals and between deeply-held personal convictions.

Media celebrities include the actors **Dan Aykroyd**, **Paddy Considine** and **Daryl Hannah**, the artists **Steven Wiltshire**, **Michael Madore** and **Peter Myers** (author of "An Exact Mind, An Artist With Asperger Syndrome"), the musicians singer-composer **Gary Numan** (in Tubeway Army and solo), singer-songwriter **Ladyhawke** (also known as Pip Brown), lead singer, songwriter and guitarist **Craig Nicholls** of The Vines and the animal-handling expert and author **Temple Grandin**, who has been the subject of many documentaries and a feature film.

B Books and websites *(Stuart Neilson)*

B.1 Further reading

This is a short collection of books with further information about the topics in the chapters of this book. We have aimed to find comprehensive books that are not over-priced, and to select a small number of representative titles that cover these topics in greater depth. There are many books about autism, often covering similar ground.

The Complete guide to Asperger's Syndrome by Tony Attwood (2007). If you had to pick only one book about Asperger syndrome, this book would be a good choice. It is expensive, but it comprehensively covers most issues from diagnosis, through symptoms to everyday life and relationships.

Autism — The Eighth Colour of the Rainbow: Learn to Speak Autistic by Florica Stone (2004). Once you get over the barrier of "unconditional love" as a component of therapy, Florica Stone provides some first class advice on conflict and resolution — most stress arises when there is a conflict between a child's behaviour and the adults' expectations. This book is limited to childhood and a few adolescence issues, and it would be wonderful to see the same practical conflict-resolution extended into adulthood.

All Cats Have Asperger Syndrome by Kathy Hoopmann (2006). You might like this book, and if so, then it is worth including here. It is a picture book containing one-page photographs of cats and kittens accompanied by short descriptions of how Asperger syndrome feels, in a form that may really help to explain your own feelings when words don't work.

Freaks, Geeks & Asperger Syndrome by Luke Jackson (2002). Don't let the title put you off reading this excellent, first-hand account of growing up with Asperger syndrome. Luke Jackson was fifteen when he wrote this guide, and it is grounded firmly in his real-life concerns of school, his Mum and his siblings.

Asperger Syndrome And Anxiety: A Guide To Successful Stress Management by Nick Dubin is one of the best books on coping with anxiety.

Survival Strategies for People on the Autism Spectrum Disorder by Marc Fleisher (2006), **Unwritten Rules Of Social Relationships** by Temple Grandin and Sean Barron, Edited by Veronica Zysk (2005) and **Asperger Syndrome and Social Relationships: Adults Speak Out about Asperger Syndrome**, edited by Genevieve Edmonds and Luke Beardon (2008) cover issues of social connections, education and employment for adults on the spectrum.

Sex, Sexuality and the Autism Spectrum by Wendy Lawson (2005) is a fairly down-to-earth user-guide to your own body and sexuality whereas **Asperger's Syndrome and Sexuality: From Adolescence through Adulthood** by Isabelle Hénault is more technical and aimed towards education and intervention.

Aspergirls: Empowering Females with Asperger Syndrome by Rudy Simone (2010) is forceful book from an older woman with Asperger syndrome.

B.2 Books written by people on the spectrum

There are several books written by people with a diagnosis of autism spectrum disorder, including:

"Urville" by Gilles Tréhin (2006) — a compilation of detailed drawings and historical, geographical, cultural and economic descriptions of an imaginary city called Urville.

Temple Grandin has written many books, including the autobiographical **"Thinking in Pictures"** (2005), **"The Unwritten Rules of Social Relationships"** (with Sean Barron, 2005) and **"The Autistic Brain: Thinking Across The Spectrum"** (with Richard Panek, 2013).

Luke Jackson's **"Freaks, Geeks & Asperger Syndrome: A User**

Guide To Adolescence" (2002) was written when he was thirteen.

Peter Myers' book **"An Exact Mind: An artist with Asperger Syndrome"** (with Simon Baron-Cohen and Sally Wheelwright, 2004) details the thinking behind and meaning for the artist of many beautifully-reproduced images of his work.

Higashida Naoki **"The Reason I Jump: The Inner Voice of a Thirteen-Year-Old Boy With Autism"** (translated by David Mitchell, 2013) is the written voice of a boy who does not speak.

Dawn Prince-Hughes describes her work as a primatologist, her growing understanding of (human and animal) relationships and her life with autism in **"Songs of the Gorilla Nation: My Journey Through Autism"** (2004).

John Elder Robison's **"Look Me in the Eye: My Life With Asperger's"** is a no-holds-barred autobiography of the difficulties of growing up with undiagnosed Asperger syndrome.

Rudy Simone in **"Aspergirls: Empowering Females with Asperger Syndrome"** (2010) and Donna Williams in **"Nobody, Nowhere"** (1994), **"Somebody, Somewhere"** (1994) and **"The Jumbled Jigsaw: An Insider's Approach to the Treatment of Autistic Spectrum 'Fruit Salads'"** (2007) describe the experience of being a woman with a condition that is strongly associated with boys and men.

Liane Holliday Willey describes her life and diagnosis — after recognizing the same traits in her own daughter — in **"Pretending to be Normal: Living with Asperger's Syndrome"** (1999).

Finally, Cindy Ariel and Robert Naseef's edited collection **"Voices from the Spectrum: Parents, Grandparents, Siblings, People with Autism, and Professionals Share their Wisdom"** (2006) offers many varied insights into autism from a range of people on the spectrum and from those who are close to them.

B.3 Internet discussions and forums

WrongPlanet (www.wrongplanet.net/ forums.html) is a very active forum for discussing almost any issue related to autism, Asperger Syndrome, ADHD, PDDs, and other neurological differences. The participants are spread throughout the world. The site also delivers well-written articles and professionally-produced videos about life with autism.

Asperger's and ASD UK Forum (www.asd-forum.org.uk/ forum/) is a UK-based discussion forum.

Spectrumites (www.spectrumites.com/) is a community and activism site focusing on autistic rights activism, connections between autistic people, and autism support. Spectrumites operates a discussion forum at www.spectrumites.com/ forums/ index.php.

AspiesCentral (www.aspiescentral.com/ forum.php) is a discussion community for people with Asperger syndrome, autism and associates.

The Thinking Person's Guide to Autism (www.thinkingautismguide.com/) aims to publish "what you need to know about autism, from autistics, professionals, and parents" and is an edited blog generated by a group of dedicated adult writers.

Autism Speaks (www.autismspeaks.org/) is one of the largest (US) charities that advocates for families affected by autism, and a major research funder. There is an official blog at www.autismspeaks.org/blog

Age of Autism (www.ageofautism.com/), which describes itself as "the daily web newspaper of the autism epidemic", is an activist site promoting the (unbalanced) argument that we are witnessing an epidemic created by vaccination, pollution, toxins and over-use of medication. It is a rapid source of political news about autism in the US.

C Organisations and services
(Stuart Neilson)

C.1 Local and national services

Aspect, AS Adult Support Service. A Cork Association for Autism Service
73 Penrose Wharf, Penrose Quay, Cork
(021) 2393678 — info@caaspect.ie
corkautism.ie/aspect/

aspire, the Asperger Syndrome Association of Ireland Limited
Coleraine House, Carmichael Centre, Coleraine Street, Dublin 7
(01) 8780027 — development@aspireireland.ie
www.aspireireland.ie/

Brothers of Charity National Office
Kilcornan House, Clarinbridge, Co. Galway
(091) 796623 — winifredohanrahan@galway.brothersofcharity.ie
www.brothersofcharity.ie/

COPE Foundation
Bonnington, Montenotte, Cork
(021) 4643100 — headoffice@cope-foundation.ie
www.cope-foundation.ie/

Cork Association for Autism (see also Aspect)
18 Cook Street, Cork
(021) 4271808 — caa@indigo.ie
corkautism.ie/

Irish Autism Action
41 Newlands, Mullingar, Co. Westmeath
(044) 9330709 — info@autismireland.ie
www.autismireland.ie/ — www.irishautismaction.blogspot.ie/ —
www.facebook.com/Irishautism

National Autistic Society (UK)
393 City Road, London, EC1V 1NG, United Kingdom

(Administrative Office)
+44 (0)20 7833 2299 — nas@nas.org.uk
www.autism.org.uk/

National Learning Network
Cootehill Road, Cavan Town, Co. Cavan
(049) 4331544 or (01) 2057313 — info@nln.ie
www.nln.ie/

Shine
The Shine Centre, 7 Weston View Ballinrea Road, Carrigaline, Co. Cork
(021) 4377052 — info@shineireland.com
www.shineireland.com/ and www.facebook.com/shine.ireland

Tuiscint Centre
Mount Pleasant Business Park, Mount Pleasant Avenue Upper, Ranelagh, Dublin 6
(01) 4911473 — tuiscint@eircom.net

C.2 Diagnosis

Joanne Douglas
Consultant Psychologist, The Spectrum Centre, 14 Northland Row, Dungannon, Co. Tyrone, BT71 6AP
+44 (0)28 8772 9810 — www.thespectrumcentre.com/

Seamus Feehan
Regional ASD Team, Marian House, Leghanamore Togher, Cork
(021) 4347087

Professor Michael Fitzgerald
Unit 3, Medical Centre, Main Street, Blanchardstown, Dublin 15
(01) 8211796 — fitzi@iol.ie — www.professormichaelfitzgerald.eu/

Dr Eimear Philbin-Bowman
Dublin Well Woman Centre, 25 Capel Street, Dublin or 67 Pembroke Road, Ballsbridge, Dublin 4
(01) 6681108 — info@wellwomancentre.ie

C.3 Third level student support services

C.3.1 Institutes of Technology

Athlone Institute of Technology: Disability Support Service
(090) 646 8142 — blangtry@ait.ie
www.ait.ie/disability/

Cork Institute of Technology: Access Service (021) 433 5107
(direct) or (021) 433 5138 (Access Service) — disability@cit.ie
www.cit.ie/ studentlife/ access_disability/ disabilities/

Dublin Institute of Technology: Disability Support Service (01)
402 7681 — disability@dit.ie
www.dit.ie/ campuslife/ disability/

Dundalk Institute of Technology: Disability and Student Quality
Office (042) 9370237 — Ciara.OShea@dkit.ie
www.dkit.ie/ student-quality

Dun Laoghaire Institute of Art Design and Technology: Access
Office
www.iadt.ie/ en/ ProspectiveStudents/ HowtoApply/ AccessOffice/

Galway-Mayo Institute of Technology: Access and Disability
Office (091) 742129 or (091) 742182 — accessoffice@gmit.ie
www.gmit.ie/ access-office/ access-and-disability-office

Institute of Technology Blanchardstown: Student Services
Office (01) 8851592 — sid@itb.ie
www.itb.ie/ CampusStudentLife/ studentservices.html

Institute of Technology Carlow: Access Office (059) 9175603 —
aisling.mchugh or (059) 9175616 — angela.costelloe
www.itcarlow.ie/ study-at-itc/ access-office.htm

Institute of Technology Sligo: Access Office — (071) 9305381
— access@itsligo.ie
itsligo.ie/ student-hub/ student-help/ student-support-services/
access-office/

Institute of Technology Tallaght: Disability Office — (01) 4042606 — garry.toner@ittdublin.ie
www.it-tallaght.ie/ index.cfm/ page/ disabilityoffice

Institute of Technology Tralee: Access Office — (066) 7191682 — valerie.moore@staff.ittralee.ie
www.ittralee.ie/ InformationFor/ CurrentStudents/ StudentLife/ StudentServices/ AccessandDisability/

Letterkenny Institute of Technology: Access Office — (074) 9186170 — brian.mcgonagle@lyit.ie
www.lyit.ie/ studentlife/ studentservices/ accessoffice/

Limerick Institute of Technology: Disability Support @ LIT — (061) 293112 — broze.odonovan@lit.ie
www.lit.ie/ Disability/ default.aspx

Waterford Institute of Technology: Disability Service — (051) 302871 — disabilityoffice@wit.ie
www.wit.ie/ current_students/ student_life_and_learning/ disability_service

C.3.2 Universities

Dublin City University: Disability & Learning Support Service — (01) 700 5927 — disability.service@dcu.ie
www.dcu.ie/ students/ disability/ index.shtml

National College of Art & Design: Disability Service — (01) 636 4314 — assistivetechnology@staff.ncad.ie
www.ncad.ie/ students/ support-services/ disability-service/

National College of Ireland: Disability Support Services — 1850 221 721
www.ncirl.ie/ Campus/ StudentServices/ DisabilitySupport.aspx

University College Cork: Disability Support Service — (021) 4902985 — dssinfo@ucc.ie
www.ucc.ie/ en/ dss/

University College Dublin: UCD Access Centre — (01) 716 7565 — disability@ucd.ie
www.ucd.ie/ disability

NUI Galway: Disability Support Service — (091) 492813 — disability.service@nuigalway.ie
www.nuigalway.ie/ student_life/ student_services/ disability_office/

NUI Maynooth: Disability Office — (01) 7086025 — access.office@nuim.ie
access.nuim.ie/ disability

Trinity College Dublin: Disability Service — (01) 8963111 — disab@tcd.ie
www.tcd.ie/ disability

University of Limerick: Disability Support Services — (061) 202700
www2.ul.ie/ web/ WWW/ Services/Student_Affairs/ Student_Specialised_Supports/ Disability_Support_Services

C.3.3 General student support websites

Quest for Learning is a European Union project to promote understanding of Open and Distance Learning (ODL) and Information and Communication Technology (ICT) for education, with information about study skills and planning.
www.questforlearning.org/

Student Finance Information provides information about financial support for further and higher education in Ireland, including the Student Grant, free fees, the Fund for Students with Disabilities, the Back to Education Allowance and the Student Assistance Fund.
www.studentfinance.ie/

Higher Education Authority provides information about policy, funding and statistics on higher education in Ireland.
www.hea.ie/ en/ students

D Glossary of terminology (Stuart Neilson)

This is a glossary of terminology and abbreviations related to autism spectrum disorder. Although we have tried to avoid using abbreviations and unnecessarily medical or technical language within this book, there are times when it is hard to avoid jargon, and times when the abbreviation is simply more commonly used than the fully-written phrase.

ABA — Applied Behaviour Analysis is a well-documented and well-validated process of intensive behaviour modification for children with autism.

ADD — See *attention-deficit disorder*

ADHD — See *attention-deficit hyperactivity disorder*

AQ — The Autism Spectrum Quotient (or AQ) test is a screening questionnaire in which a higher score indicates a greater probablity of "clinically significant levels of autistic traits". Online versions have appeared in a number of places, including Wired magazine www.wired.com/ wired/ archive/ 9.12/ aqtest.html

AS — See *Asperger syndrome*

ASD — See *autism spectrum disorder*

Asperger syndrome (AS) — A specific diagnosis within the group *autism spectrum disorder* that has evolved a distinct identity from *high-functioning autism* (HFA). There is debate about whether Asperger syndrome is biologically distinct from other forms of autism.

attention-deficit disorder (ADD) — A subtype of *ADHD* in which inattentiveness predominates and in which hyperactivity and impulsiveness are not pronounced.

attention-deficit hyperactivity disorder (ADHD) — A neurobehavioural disorder involving inattentiveness, hyperactivity and impulsiveness.

autism spectrum disorder (ASD) — a group of neurodevelopmental conditions classed as a pervasive developmental disorders (PDD). Autism spectrum disorders are characterised by the "triad of impairments": social deficits, communication difficulties and stereotyped or repetitive behaviours and interests.

CAMHS — The Child and Adolescent Mental Health Service is a referral-based service for children and adolescents that is a body responsible for children with autism who have needs separate from education, before and throughout school age. There is some overlap with both education and disability services. The charity Reach Out describes the services available at ie.reachout.com/ getting-help/ face-to-face-help/ services-explained/ child-and-adolescent-mental-health-services/

CAO — The Central Applications Office is the centralised system for processing applications to the first year of undergraduate courses at higher education institutes in Ireland, www.cao.ie/. The CAO does not make decisions about accepting or rejecting students, which is still done by each institution independently. DARE, the Disability Access Route to Education, provides reduced-points access for students with disabilities — see *DARE*.

CBT — Cognitive Behavioural Therapy is a talking therapy that encourages people to challenge difficult thoughts and behaviours, with proven effectiveness in treating anxiety, depression, eating disorders (anorexia and bulimia) and OCD. CBT is both the first line (before medication) and preferred therapy for most of these mood-related conditions.

Concerta — See *methylphenidate*

DARE — The Disability Access Route to Education (DARE) is a college and university admissions scheme which offers places on a reduced points basis to school leavers under 23 years old with disabilities. www.accesscollege.ie/ dare/ index.php

DBT — Dialectical Behaviour Therapy combines CBT and Mindfulness therapies and may be a particular counsellor's approach to talking therapy.

DNA — Deoxyribose nucleic acid, the molecular content of our genes.

DSM — The American Psychiatric Association's Diagnostic and Statistical Manual of Mental Disorders, one of the primary reference guides for diagnosis. Autism was first included as "infantile autism" 1980 (revised to "autistic disorder" in 1987) in DSM-III, then within the pervasive developmental disorders in DSM-IV in 1994. The DSM-5 (May 2013) combines autism, Asperger syndrome and pervasive developmental disorder, not otherwise specified (PDD-NOS) within a single diagnostic category of Autism Spectrum Disorder.

dyscalculia — A learning disability involving difficulty understanding or learning mathematics. Dyscalculia affects people across the entire intelligence range. www.sess.ie/ categories/ specific-learning-disabilities/ dyscalculia

dyslexia — A learning disability involving difficulty understanding, reading or writing text. Dyslexia affects people across the entire intelligence range. www.sess.ie/ categories/ specific-learning-disabilities/ dyslexia

EBT — Employer-based training combining further education with on-the-job training, often associated with enhanced welfare allowances.

empathy — The ability to recognise, identify and respond to emotions — of other people and yourself. Cognitive empathy (theory of mind) describes the ability to identify mental states, whereas affective empathy describes the ability to respond appropriately. People with autism have impaired cognitive empathy (fail to recognize emotion, in themselves or others) but unimpaired affective empathy (will feel the appropriate emotion once it is understood).

EPSEN — The Education for Persons with Special Educational

Needs Act 2004, which defines the rights to an educational assessment, a statement of special needs and an action plan. www.irishstatutebook.ie/ 2004/ en/ act/ pub/ 0030/ print.html

executive function — A collection of processes involving problem-solving, task management and responding to unexpected change (or interruption) that are impaired in autism. Executive function can be supplemented with good planning and effective note-taking.

FÁS — the Employment and Training Authority or Foras Áiseanna Saothair (www.fas.ie/ en/), which means 'growth' in Irish.

GFCF — A gluten-free, casein-free diet eliminates all gluten (occurring naturally in wheat, rye and barley, and by contamination in oats) and all casein (dairy protein). The diet is widely used with children with autism, although many bodies (including the The American Academy of Pediatrics, the Cochrane Collaboration and NICE) have concluded that there is no compelling evidence for the diet — except in children with confirmed coeliac disease. Some peole also exclude soya and soya-contaminated produce, the GFCFSF diet.

GP — The General Practitioner is the first point of contact for many services, including non-medical services (such as welfare-related benefits). Access to psychiatric and educational assessment is by referral from a GP or other front-line professional.

gravitational insecurity — Fear or nervousness associated with balance and underactive vestibular processing, which can lead to caution with heights, swinging motions or climbing. It is notable that some people with vestibular dysfunction react positively to vestibular stimulation and enjoying swinging, spinning and other motion. Gravitational insecurity is associated with *Sensory Processing Disorder*.

HEA — The Higher Education Authority (www.hea.ie/) is the statutory body responsible for planning and policy for third-level education in Irish universities, institutes of technology and some other third-level institutes.

HFA — See *high-functioning autism*

high-functioning autism (HFA) — A diagnosis that is frequently made for people with autism who have no cognitive deficits. HFA is usually diagnosed earlier than Asperger syndrome, and some clinicians argue that the two conditions are otherwise indistinguishable.

HR — Human Resources is the department of an organisation responsible for recruitment, training and discipline of employees — also called a Personnel Department.

HSE — The Health Service Executive of Ireland, hse.ie/ eng/

hyper- — A prefix meaning elevated, raised or excessive.

hyperacusis — Excessively sensitive hearing in which noise can be unpleasant or painful, with defensive responses such as wearing ear-muffs (in any weather), covering the ears or moving away.

hypersensitive — Excessively sensitive in one of the principal five senses (sight, hearing, touch, smell or taste) or the lesser known three senses (vestibular, proprioceptive and interoceptive).

hypervigilance — A state of heightened sensory arousal accompanied by anxiety and behaviours associated with detecting threats, such as monitoring the environment for changes, movement or fearful stimuli. Hypervigilance is tiring.

hypo- — A prefix meaning lowered, reduced or inadequate.

hyposensitive — Under-responsive in one of the principal five senses (sight, hearing, touch, smell or taste) or the lesser known three senses (vestibular, proprioceptive and interoceptive).

IBS — Irritable bowel syndrome is a symptomatic diagnosis based on function gastrointestinal disorder, usually diarrhoea or constipation (which may alternate) and pain or discomfort. Despite affecting perhaps 10% of the population and causing great distress, there is no identifiable organic cause. Soluble fibre, dietary changes and symtomatic relief of spasm and pain may help some people.

ICD — The World Health Organisation's International Classification of Disease, www.who.int/ classifications/ icd/ en/.

interoception — In addition to the usual 'five senses' (hearing, sight, smell, taste and touch), humans also feel internal sensations from our circulatory system, lungs, digestive tract, bladder and bowel. Over-responsive interoception causes discomfort, whereas under-responsiveness might be associated with bladder or bowel dysfunction.

Methylin — See *methylphenidate*

methylphenidate — (branded as Concerta, Methylin, Ritalin) A psychostimulant drug prescribed for ADHD / ADD and used to maintain alertness and attention.

MRI — Magnetic Resonance Imaging is a technique for examining structures inside the body, including brain-imaging. MRI does not carry the same risks as X-Ray imaging and provides greater detail. There may be structural brain differences in people with autism that could, one day, lead to better diagnosis and evaluation.

NICE — The UK National Institute for Health and Care Excellence is one of the leading authorities on health care provision, with Clinical Guidance documents on autism recognition and intervention (publications.nice.org.uk/ autism-recognition-referral-diagnosis-and-management-of-adults -on-the-autism-spectrum-cg142).

NIMH — The US National Institute of Mental Health (www.nimh.nih.gov/ health/ topics/ autism-spectrum-disorders-pervasive-developmental-disorders/ index.shtml) is one of the leading authorities on development and well-being, with reputable information about autism recognition and intervention.

NLN — The National Learning Network (www.nln.ie/) is the largest non-Government training organisation in Ireland.

NT — NeuroTypical is a term coined by people with autism to define people without autism, and later to define people without any atypical neurology (such as developmental conditions, dyslexia, ADHD or learning impairments).

obsessive-compulsive disorder (OCD) — An anxiety-driven behaviour in which someone obsessively follows routines or repeats actions to ease the sense of anxiety. *Perseveration* and restricted and repetitive behaviours are a part of autism, although often without apparent anxiety.

OCD — See *obsessive-compulsive disorder*

OTC — See *over-the-counter drug*

over-the-counter (OTC) drug — Over-the-counter medications are drugs which can be bought from a pharmacy without a prescription, although some (such as pain medication) is sold in limited quantities and after questioning about symptoms.

pervasive developmental disorder — A group of five diagnostic categories within the DSM-IV that includes the specific diagnoses of autism, Asperger syndrome, childhood disintegrative disorder and Rett syndrome, and the non-specific diagnosis of pervasive developmental disorder, not otherwise specified (PDD-NOS). PDD-NOS is the most common diagnosis.

PDD — See *pervasive developmental disorder*

PDD-NOS — Pervasive developmental disorder, not otherwise specified. Within the DSM-IV diagnostic criteria, this is a pervasive developmental disorder that does not meet the criteria for one of the specific developmental disorders of autism, Asperger syndrome, childhood disintegrative disorder or Rett syndrome. PDD-NOS is the most frequently diagnosed pervasive developmental disorder.

PEG — Polyethylene glycol (as the prescription-only medication Movicol) is an osmotic laxative that draws moisture into the gastrointestinal tract to soften the bowel contents and relieve constipation. It is found to be gentler and more effective than either non-soluble fibre bulking agents or stimulant-irritant laxatives such as senna extract, especially in chronic constipation associated with IBS.

perseveration — The perseverance with behaviours and thoughts that are linked with a narrow range of interests, or a single focus of interest. A strong focus and drive only becomes "perseveration" when other people decide that the focus is not important enough or the focus is excessive by their standards.

PMR — Progressive muscle relaxation is a method for managing tension than can be an effective intervention for stress, anxiety and persistent headaches or pain. The exercise may consist of tensing and then relaxing each muscle group — from the tips of the toes to the scalp — while in a comfortable place, or it may also involve visual imagery. PMR is most effective when practised regularly, with benefits that extend to managing anxiety in public places.

proprioception — A sense of your own body within the local environment, or the parts of your body in relation to each other. At the simplest level, proprioception helps you to safely cut things that you are holding with your hand, even when you can't see your fingers, or to bring a fork to your mouth. At a more complex level, it helps you coordinate walking and avoiding obstacles.

PRSI — Pay Related Social Insurance is a system for collecting social and health insurance taken directly from income (in the same way as tax is deducted) and used to fund social welfare and pension payments. Sufficient PRSI credits are required in order to qualify for benefits that are not means-tested.

Ritalin — See *methylphenidate*

Restricted and repetitive behaviours — Stereotyped and repeated actions, or interests that are pursued to an obsessive degree (i.e. to the extent of limiting quality of life). Some apparently 'non-functional' RRBs and rituals have significance and value to the individual pursuing them.

RRB — see *restricted and repetitive behaviours*

self-harm — Deliberate acts that cause injury (including cutting, scratching, biting or hitting yourself) and behaviours around food-control (anorexia and bulimia). Self-harm can act as a form of self-comforting and as an expression of control over mental and emotional distress. Self-harm can be divided into behaviours that have no fatal intent and those that are related to suicide or expressions of suicidal thoughts, for which you should seek urgent help.

self-medication — Using *over-the-counter* drugs, supplements or other substances (legal and illegal) to treat conditions or discomfort that is undiagnosed or is not responding to prescribed treatments. Common self-medications behaviours include the beneficial (diet, exercise and some food supplements), relatively harmless (ineffective supplements or therapies) and the harmful (overuse of pain medication, alcohol, cannabis and other drugs).

SEN — Special educational needs.

Sensory Processing Disorder — Sometimes also called sensory integration dysfunction or SPD is a term pioneered by occupational therapist Dr Anna Jean Ayres. Although SPD is not recognized by all practitioners, there are reports that appropriate occupational therapy improves sensory integration, coordination, tactile sensitivity, anxiety and other signs of poor neurological integration of the senses.

SNRI — Serotonin-norepinephrine reuptake inhibitor are antidepressant drugs that are also used to treat ADHD, OCD, and some forms of chronic pain.

SSRI — Selective serotonin re-uptake inhibitors are antidepressant drugs that are also used to treat generalised anxiety disorder and OCD.

STEM — In education the Science, Technology, Engineering and Mathematics fields are often seen as a separate stream from the arts, humanities and (sometimes) the life sciences. STEM skills are typically spatial ability, logic and maths rather than language skills. Students can be pressured to choose between either the STEM or the arts and humanities, largely by stereotypes hanging on one specific ability (such as arithmetic).

synaesthesia — A fascinating neurological condition in which one sense triggers another, for instance seeing numbers in colour, tasting words or smelling shapes. Some synaesthetes produce art expressing their experience of connected senses. www.uksynaesthesia.com/

tactile defensiveness — A form of sensory defensiveness to minimise the discomfort from things touching the skin, such as rough textures, wetness or light contact with passers-by. Deep-tissue pressure may be comforting. Typical signs of tactile defensiveness are wearing inappropriately long or thick clothes, or attempting to 'rub out' light touches.

task-switching — Task-switching is an important *executive function* required to complete a planned task, respond to interruptions and manage unexpected outcomes. Task-switching requires a *working memory* of the interrupted and the new tasks, as well as executive function skills to plan a new course of action.

vestibular function — The vestibular system, a fluid-filled labyrinth in the ear, provides both a sense of balance (our sense of 'up') and a sense of motion, and is associated with alertness and attention.

VHI — The Voluntary Health Insurance Board that is a statutory corporation with members are appointed by the Minister for Health, trading under the name Vhi Healthcare (www.vhi.ie/) as Ireland's biggest health insurer.

working memory — Working memory is a limited capacity to hold and manipulate information related to immediate functions, and greater working memory leads to greater *executive function*, the ability to carry out a plan and respond to change. Working memory can be very effectively supplemented with written instructions and images.

About the authors

Stuart Neilson and Diarmuid Heffernan

Stuart Neilson was diagnosed with Asperger syndrome in 2009 at the age of 45, after many years of ineffective psychiatric treatment. He has been teaching and researching at third level since 1987. He lectured in statistics at Brunel University for eight years, where he was also director of medical information systems in the Centre for the Study of Health, Sickness and Disablement. He has also lectured in medical statistics, has been involved in a variety of research projects and published extensively in international neurological journals. He has co-authored three books on multiple sclerosis and motor neuron disease. His first degree is in computer science and he has a doctorate in mathematical modelling of inherent susceptibility to fatal disease.

Diarmuid Heffernan has worked for six years supporting adults on the autistic spectrum. He has published articles about autism in peer-reviewed journals. He has considerable experience in a variety of social care fields including supporting adults with intellectual disabilities, homeless adults and teaching adolescents in a Youth Encounter Project. He has also attained a diploma in Community Development, a degree in Social Science Youth and Community, a master's degree in Social Policy and a postgraduate certificate in Teaching and Learning in Higher Education.

8172243R00140

Printed in Great Britain
by Amazon.co.uk, Ltd.,
Marston Gate.